LAST MINUTE HISTOLOGY

HISTOLOGY MADE EASY FOR MEDICAL AND NURSING STUDENTS

SIVAJITH P R

DEDICATED TO MY PARENTS, BROTHER,TEACHERS, FRIENDS AND SPECIAL DEDICATION TO LORD KRISHNA

Contents

CHAPTER I

MUSCLE TISSUE

- Muscular tissue is responsible for movement of various parts of the body.
- Comprises of elongated cells called fibres.
- They are of 3 types: Skeletal, Smooth & Cardiac

Smooth Muscle

- Non striated
- Spindle or fusiform shaped with a central oval elongated nucleus.
- Sarcoplasm contains actin & myosin filaments without an orderly arrangement. Hence only longitudinal arrangements are seen.
- Found in walls of visceral organ
- Innervated by parasympathetic & sympathetic nerve

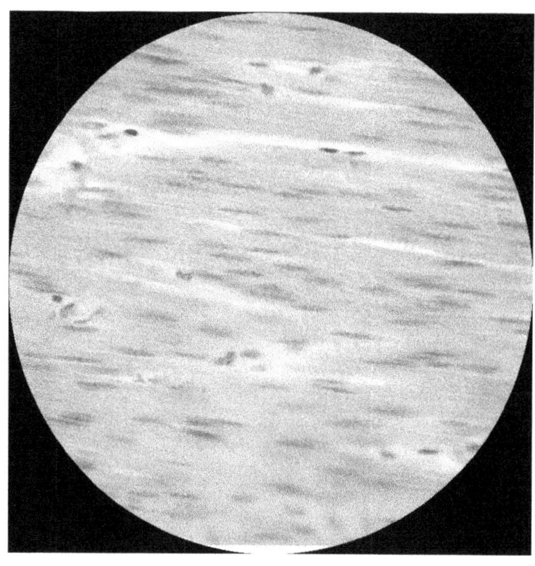

H&E SLIDES SMOOTH MUSCLE

Cardiac muscle

Are small and cylindrical compared to skeletal muscles.

Nuclei - Central , Singular & Oval (non multinucleated)

Intercalated disc between muscle fibre junctions.

INTERCALATED DISC :

Intercalated disc consist of 3 cell junctions :

- Desmosomes
- Gap junctions
- Tight junctions.

NOTE: THE PRESENCE OF INTERCALATED DISC MAKES CARDIAC MUSCLE A "FUNCTIONAL SYNCYTIUM "

Cardiac muscles are also striated but striations are not visible in low magnification

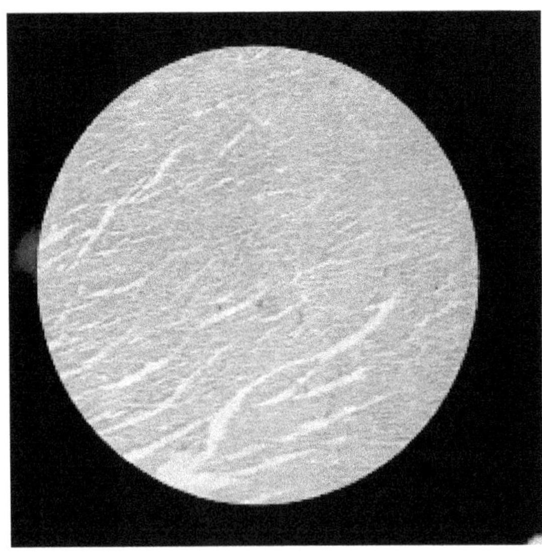

H&E SLIDES CARDIAC MUSCLE

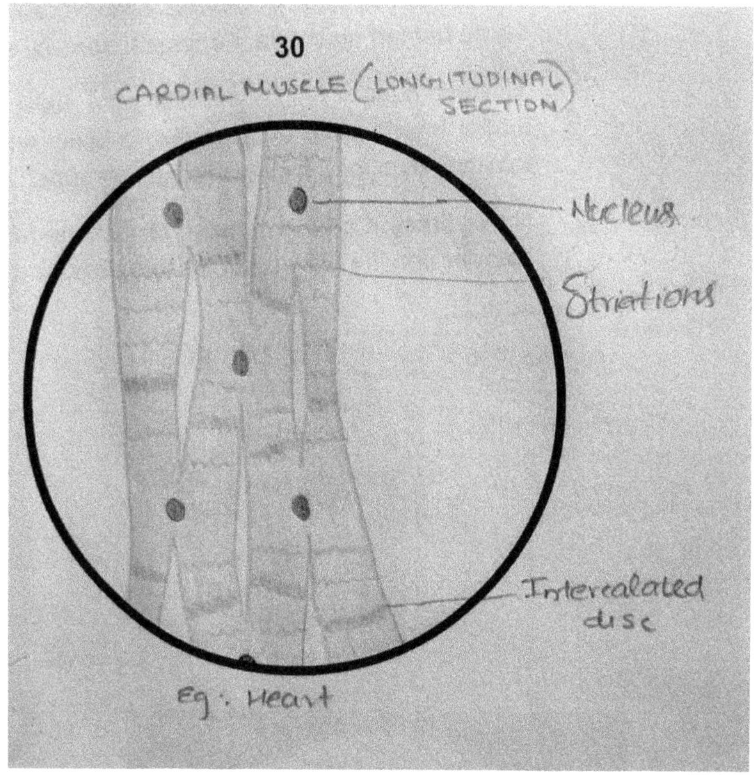

HAND MADE DIAGRAM OF CARDIAC MUSCLE

Skeletal Muscle

(eg: Muscles of limb & trunk)

[Each muscle fibre(cell) is long and cylindrical without branching.They are multinucleated with peripheral nuclei.Has Dark and Light transverse striations.]

Covering of skeletal muscles

*epimysium - covers entire muscle

*perimysium- covers muscle bundle
*endomysium - covers each fibre
*sarcolemma - cell membrane

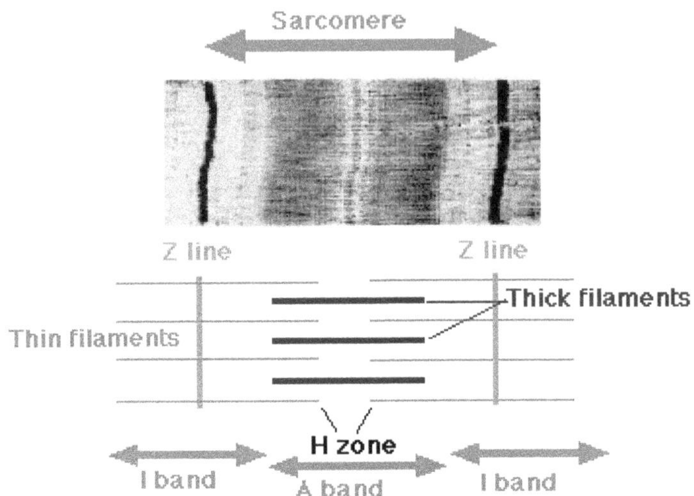

IMG: SARCOMERE

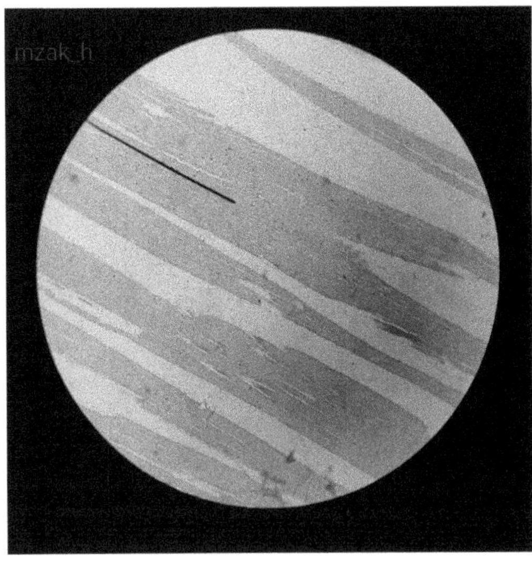

H&E SLIDES SKELETAL MUSCLE

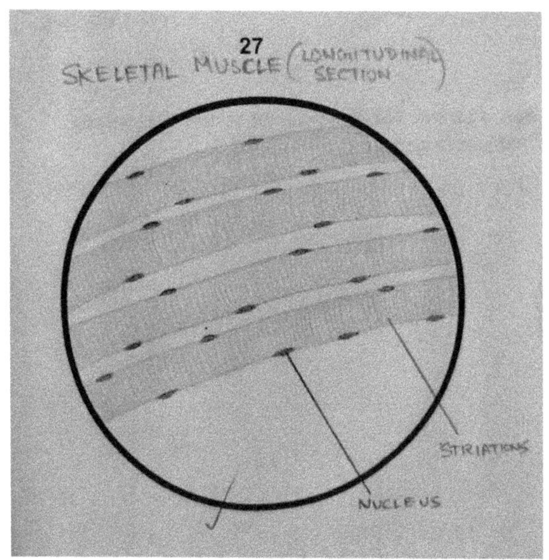

HAND MADE DIAGRAM OF SKELETAL MUSCLE

• • •

CHAPTER II

SALIVARY GLANDS

SECRETION : Saliva.

In humans there are 3 major pairs of salivary glands they are:

- PAROTID
- SUBMANDIBULAR
- SUBLINGUAL

FEATURES OF SALIVARY GLAND

°It possesses a connective tissue capsule

°This connective tissue capsule send septa, which divides the glandular parenchyma into lobes and lobules

°Each lobule contain-

*DRAINING DUCTS and

*ACINI {SECRETORY UNIT}:

They are of 3 types:

SEROUS ACINI

- Small with narrow lumen
- Lined by pyramid cells with round basal nucleus.Shows "Biphasic staining" with H&E because apical part of serous cells contain Zymogen granules which stains eosinophilic, whereas basal part take basophilic staining.

MUCOUS ACINI

- Large with wide lumen.
- Lined by Columnar cells with flattened basal nuclei.
- Apical part of mucous cells is filled with pale-staining mucous droplets.As mucus does not take stain cells look empty.

SEROMUCOUS ACINI

- Contain both Serous and Mucous acini

SALIVARY DUCT SYSTEM

°Acini opens into the Intercalated duct.

°Intercalated ducts unite to form Striated ducts , both Intercalated and Striated ducts are "Interlobular".

°These excretory ducts unite to form the main duct.

*Striated ducts are Striated because they have basal infoldings of plasma membrane and longitudinal orientation of mitochondria between these infoldings which gives the striated appearance.

MUCOUS SALIVARY GLAND (SUBLINGUAL SALIVARY GLAND)

*Characterized by a large number of mucous acini .

*Poorly developed duct system.

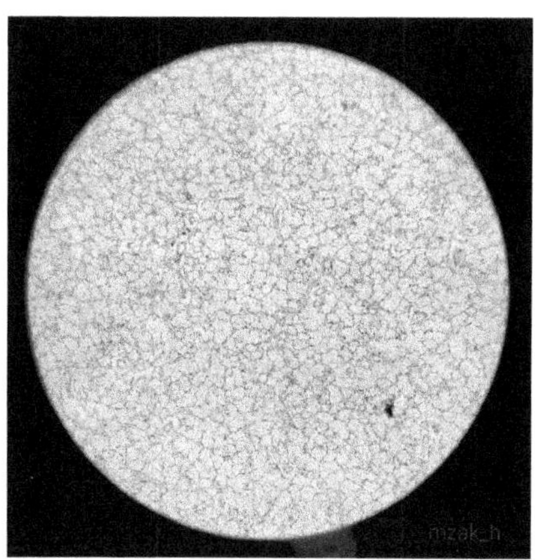

MUCOUS SALIVARY GLAND

SEROUS SALIVARY GLAND
(PAROTID SALIVARY GLAND)

*Large number of serous acini .

*Well developed duct system.

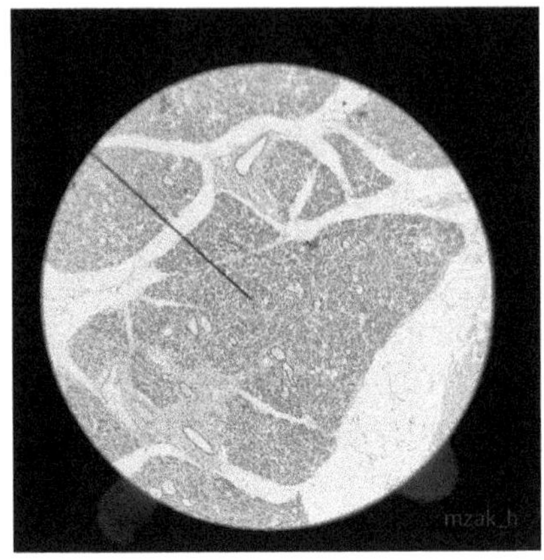

SEROUS SALIVARY GLAND

MIXED SALIVARY GLAND
(SUBMANDIBULAR SALIVARY GLAND)
*Presence of both Serous and Mucous acinus.
*Presence of "serous Demilune".
*Moderately developed duct system

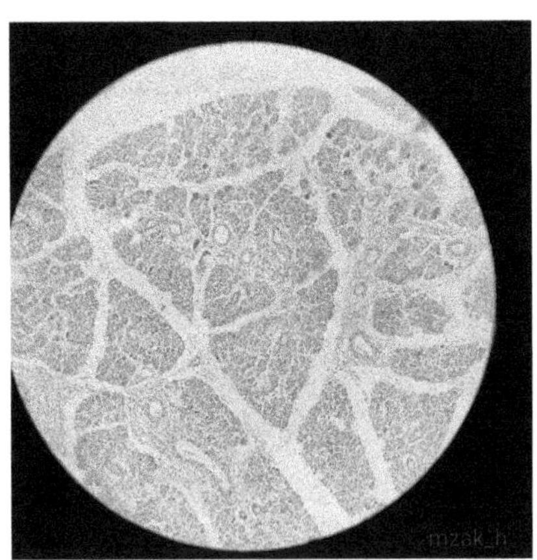

MIXED SALIVARY GLAND

• • •

CHAPTER III

PANCREAS

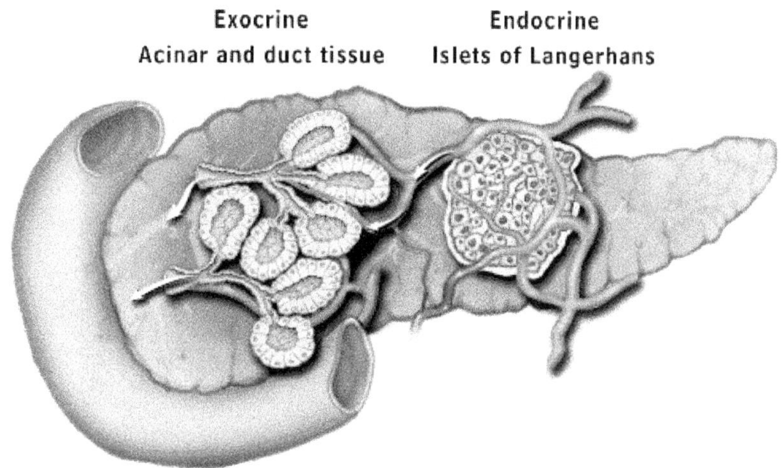

img: pancreas _ (img credit:By http://www.pancreapedia.org/reviews/pancreatogenic-type-3c-diabetes, CC BY-SA 4.0, https://en.wikipedia.org/w/index.php?curid=51023674)

Pancreas is an exo-endocrine gland, meaning,it has both exocrine and endocrine parts. Pancreas has a thick capsule, septa from this capsule divides the gland into lobules.

Exocrine part of pancreas

Exocrine part of pancreas consist of serous acini, which shows biphasic staining (refer: 'types of acini' in Salivary gland)

Some of the acini exhibits pale staining cuboidal 'centroacinar cells' within the lumen.

They represent the 'intra-acinar' part of the intercalated duct.

Endocrine part of pancreas

Consist of lightly stained 'Islets of Langerhans'

Islets of Langerhans consist of polyhedral cells which are of three types:

i. Alpha (α)
ii. Beta (β)
iii. Delta (δ)

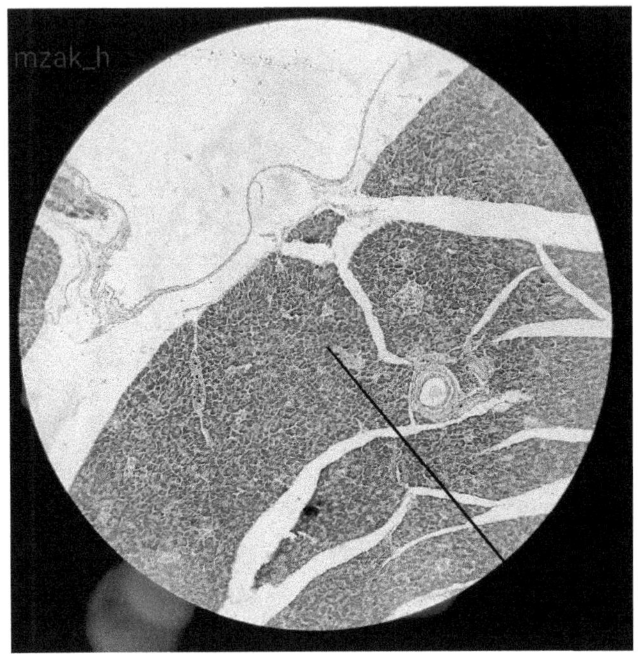

H&E SLIDE PANCREAS

• • •

CHAPTER IV

ESOPHAGUS

has four layers:

MUCOSA

- Lined by non keratinized stratified columnar epithelium.
- Lamina propria is made up of loose connective tissue.
- Muscularis mucosa has outer longitudinal and inner circular smooth muscle layers.

SUBMUCOSA

- Contains blood vessels, nerves, lymphatics and mucus secreting oesophageal glands.

MUSCULARIS EXTERNA

- Upper 1/3 is composed of skeletal muscles.
- Middle 1/3 consist of both skeletal and smooth muscles.
- Lower 1/3 is composed of purely smooth muscles.

SEROSA/ADVENTITIA

- Consist of fibrous tissue

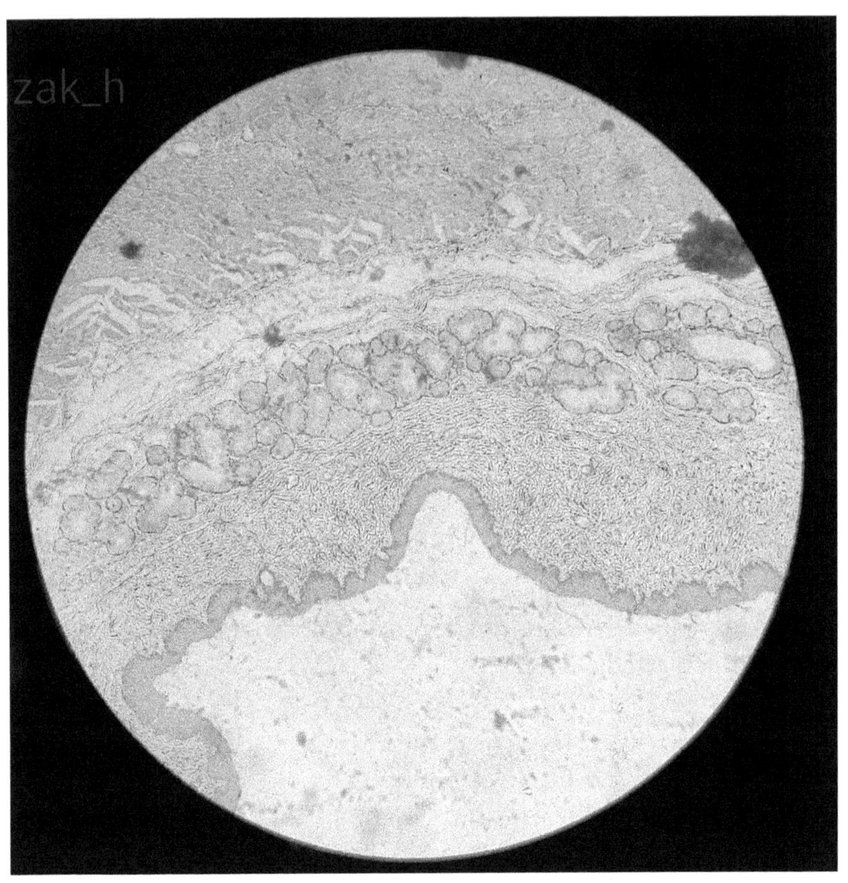

H&E SLIDE ESOPHAGUS

• • •

CHAPTER V

HISTOLOGY OF STOMACH

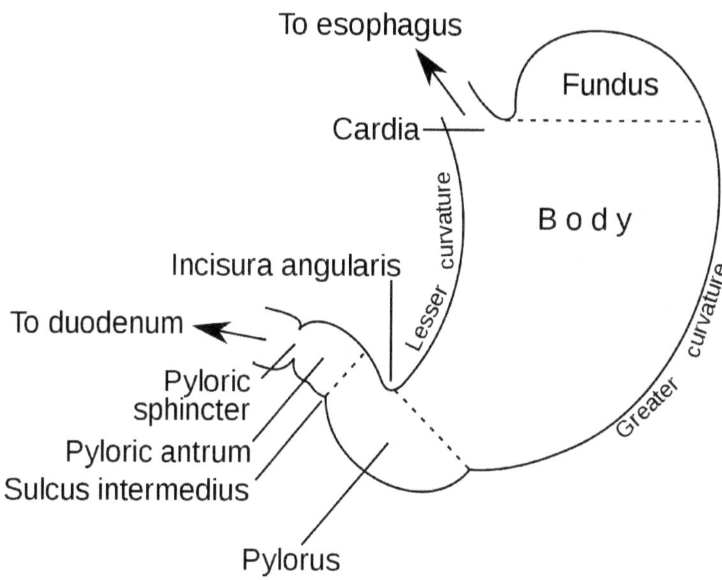

IMAGE; PARTS OF STOMACH - H.V CARTER

Stomach Fundus

Mucosa is thick and thrown into prominent folds called "rugae". It is lined by simple columnar epithelium, which invaginates into lamina propria to form gastric pits.

Lamina propria contain a large number of tubular glands, which open into gastric pits.

These glands are oriented perpendicular to the surface.

These tubular glands contain three types of cells :

- Zymogen / Chief / Peptic cells
- Parietal / Oxyntic cells

- Goblet cells

Muscularis mucosa - It is thin and made up of inner circular and outer longitudinal smooth muscle layers.

Muscularis externa - consists of inner oblique, middle ,circular, and outer longitudinal layers of smooth muscle.

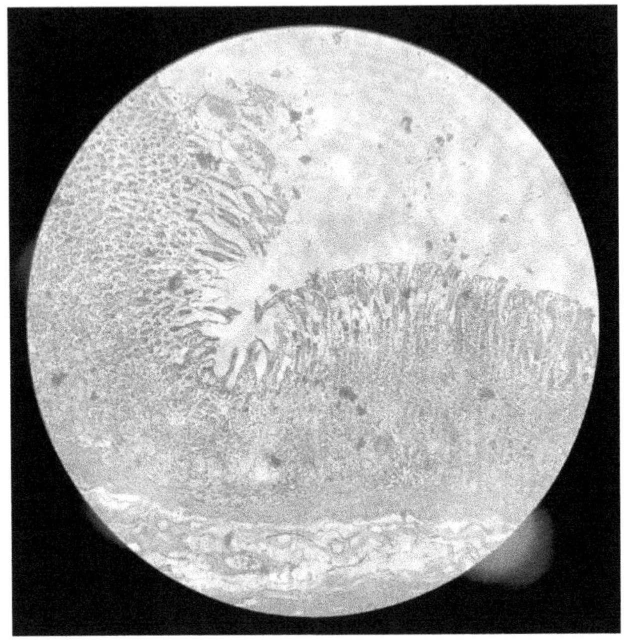

H&E SLIDE FUNDUS

Pylorus Of Stomach

MUCOSA

Lined by simple columnar epithelium. Mucous of pylorus shows gastric pits which are deeper and occupy 2/3 rd of thickness of mucosa.

LAMINA PROPRIA

Filled with glands called pyloric glands, which consists of mucous secreting cells and few parietal cells.

SUBMUCOSA

Composed of loose connective tissues.

MUSCULARIS EXTERNA

Same as that of fundus

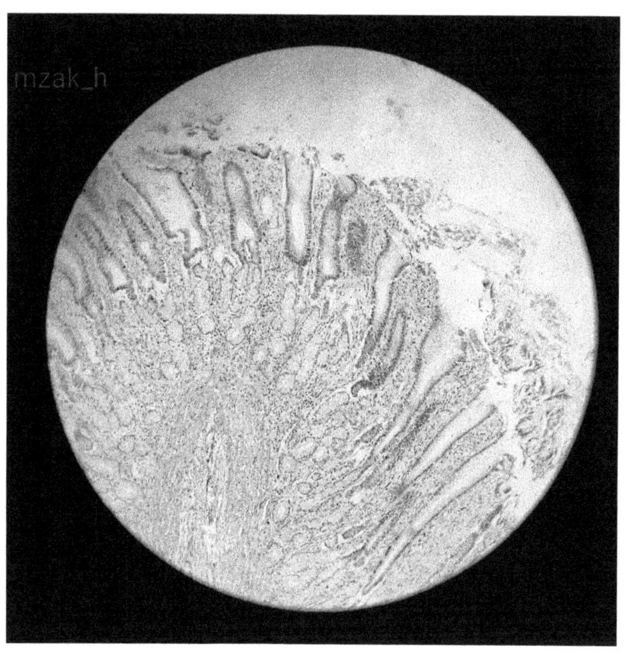

H&E SLIDE PYLORUS

• • •

CHAPTER VI

SMALL INTESTINE

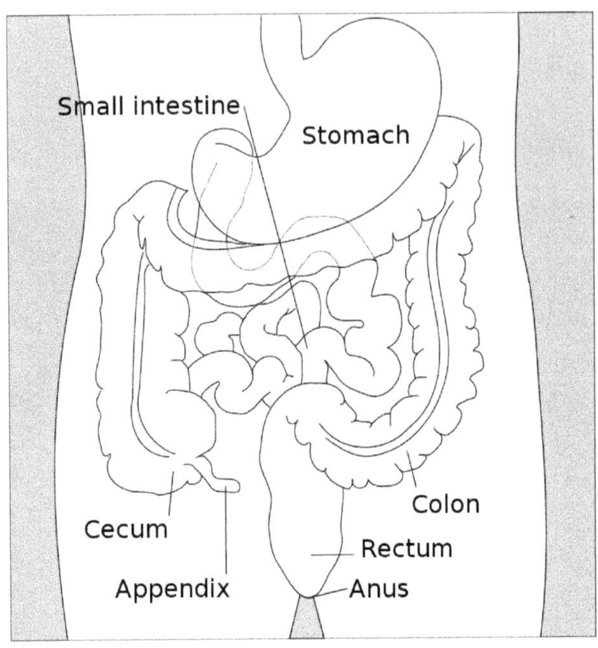

IMG; HUMAN DIGESTIVE SYSTEM _IMAGE CREDIT:Indolences created it on the English Wikipedia

Small intestine is divided into three:
1.duodenum
2.jejunum
3.ileum

DUODENUM

- It has four layers:

1. mucosa

2. bsubmucosa
3. muscularis
4. serosa

- Muscularis and serosa/adventitia layers are the same as that of the general structure of the alimentary canal. The duodenal mucosa is lined by simple columnar cells (also known as "enterocytes") and goblet cells
- In duodenum, mucosa is thrown into finger-like folds called "villi".
- Each villi has a core of lamina propria with a central lacteal and blood vessels.
- Lamina propria layers of duodenum is filled with "intestinal glands"called crypts of lieberkuhn.Crypts of lieberkuhn contain the following cells:

1. Goblet cell-mucus secreting
2. Enterocytes-they are absorptive columnar epithelium
3. Paneth cells-they lie in the deeper part of crypt they contain eosinophilic secreting granules,their exact function is unknown
4. enteroendocrine(enterochromaffin cells)-secrete substances like histamine.They possess granules which are stained by silver salt.

- The submucosa of duodenum is made up of loose connective tissue. It contains

1. blood vessels
2. tubulo-alveolar mucous glands called "brunner's gland'

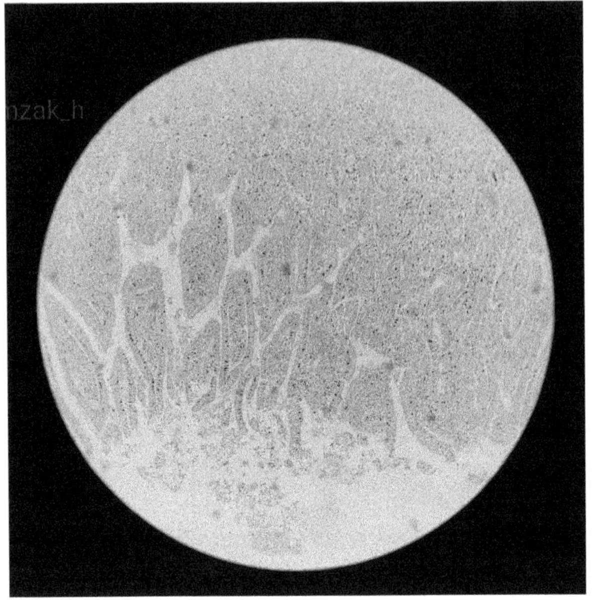

H&E SLIDE: DUODENUM

JEJUNUM

- Jejunal villi are longer and more irregular (characteristic feature)
- Muscularis mucosa is sparse or even absent.
- There are circular folds called "plicae circulares" or “valves of kerckring" which are formed by mucosa and submucosa and are permanent structures. They are absent in the first few centimetres of duodenum and distal of ileum. They are developed in jejunum.
- There are no glands in the submucosa.
- Other structures are the same as that of duodenum.

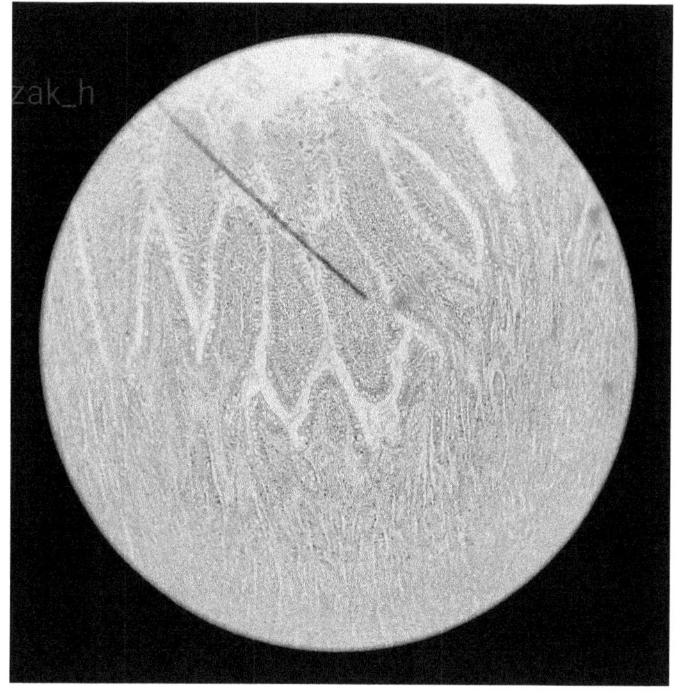

H&E SLIDE: JEJUNUM

ILEUM

- Here villi are more leaf-like.
- There are large aggregations of lymphatic tissue in the lamina propria which are known as peyer's patches.
- They contain germinal centers and are an important part of the lymphatic system.
- Other features are similar with that of duodenum and jejunum.

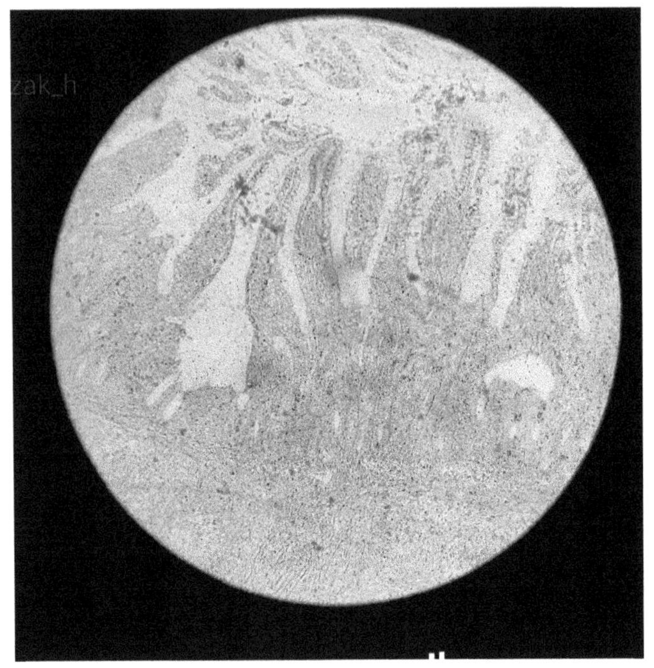

H&E SLIDE ILEUM

• • •

CHAPTER VII

LARGE INTESTINE (COLON)

- Mucosa is lined by simple columnar cells with microvilli and goblet cells.
- Goblet cells are abundant in mucosa.
- There is no villi.
- Lamina propria (of mucosa) is filled with intestinal glands (crypts of lieberkuhn).
- Muscularis mucosa is made up of inner circular and outer longitudinal layers of smooth muscles.
- Submucosa is composed of loose connective and contains blood vessels, lymphatics, nerve fibres.
- Muscularis externa - composed of inner circular and outer longitudinal smooth muscle layers.Outer longitudinal layer thickens to form "taenia coli"

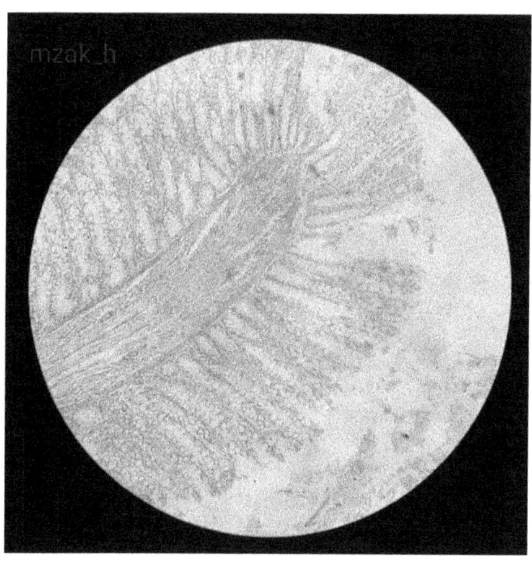

H&E SLIDE COLON

CHAPTER VIII

APPENDIX (ABDOMINAL TONSIL)

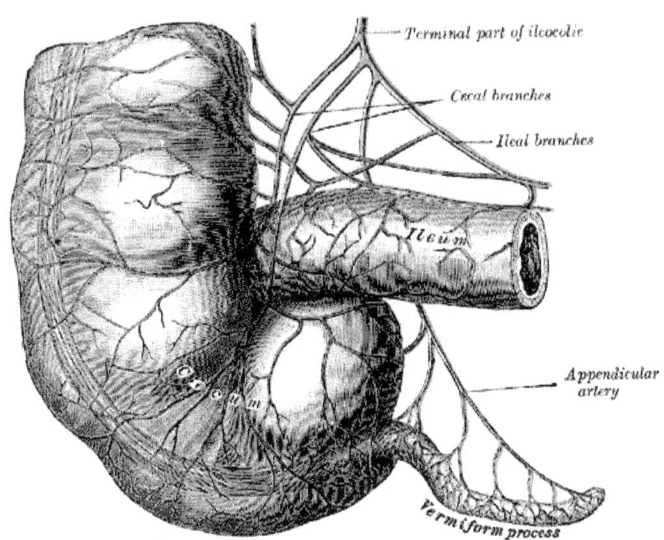

IMG: VERMIFORM APPENDIX _IMG CREDIT H.V CARTER (GRAYS ANATOMY)

❖ 4 layers:

1. Mucosa
2. Submucosa
3. Muscularis
4. Serosa

❖MUCOSA

- lined by simple columnar cells with numerous goblet cells
- devoid of villi
- crypts of lieberkuhn are few and short
- muscularis mucosa is disrupted by lymphatic follicles

❖SUBMUCOSA

- contain a ring of large lymphatic follicles with germinal centers,

  hence the name "Abdominal Tonsil."

❖MUSCULARIS EXTERNA

- consist of outer longitudinal and inner circular muscle layers.

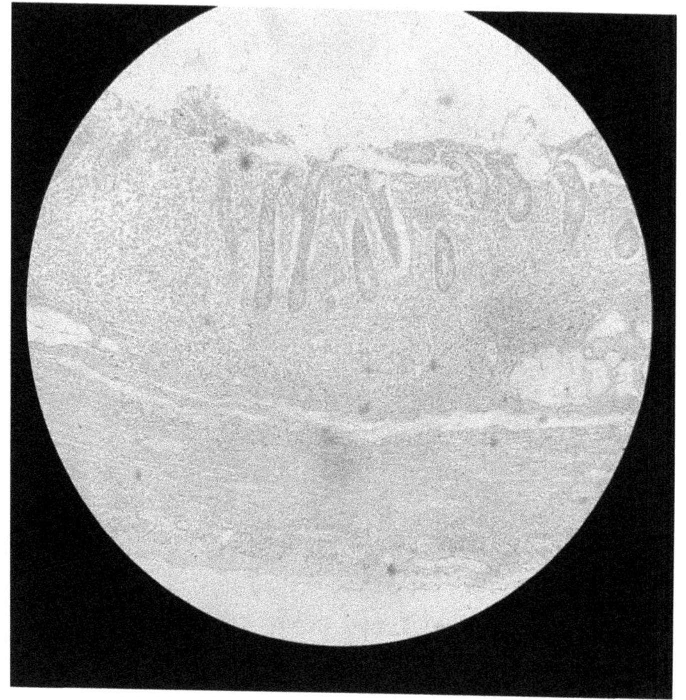

H&E SLIDES APPENDIX

• • •

CHAPTER IX

LIVER

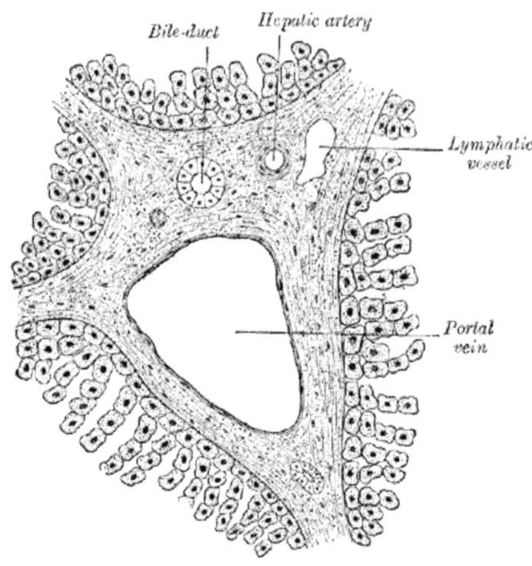

img; portal triad (img credit: By Henry Gray (1918) Anatomy of the Human Body)

- Liver is completely invested (covered) by a fibrous capsule called glisson's capsule that lies deep to the peritoneal covering of the liver.
- This glisson's capsule is thickened at porta hepatis and sends trabeculae into the interior of the liver and divides the liver parenchyma into incomplete lobules.
- These trabeculae which carry branches of hepatic artery, portal vein, hepatic duct and lymphatics is known as portal tract or portalcanal.
- Liver lobules are the structural unit of the liver.They are hexagonal in shape.
- A liver lobule consist of following structures

i. It has a central vein
ii. hepatocytes which are arranged in one cell thick plates

iii. sinusoids - Irregular spaces b/w hepatic plates are occupied by liver sinusoids.Which Are lined by discontinuous fenestrated endothelial cells.

- Some endothelial cells that line sinusoids are modified to become phagocytic kupffer cells.Sinusoids are filled with mixed arterial and venous blood from hepatic artery and portal vein.
- Sinusoids are separated from underlying plates of hepatocytes by perisinusoidal space of Disse

Note : portal vein, hepatic artery, hepatic duct together known as portal triads.

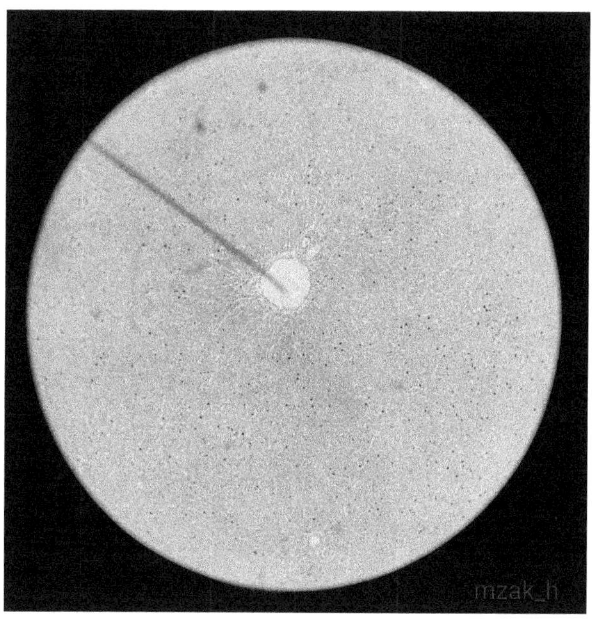

H&E SLIDE LIVER

• • •

CHAPTER X

LYMPHOID TISSUE

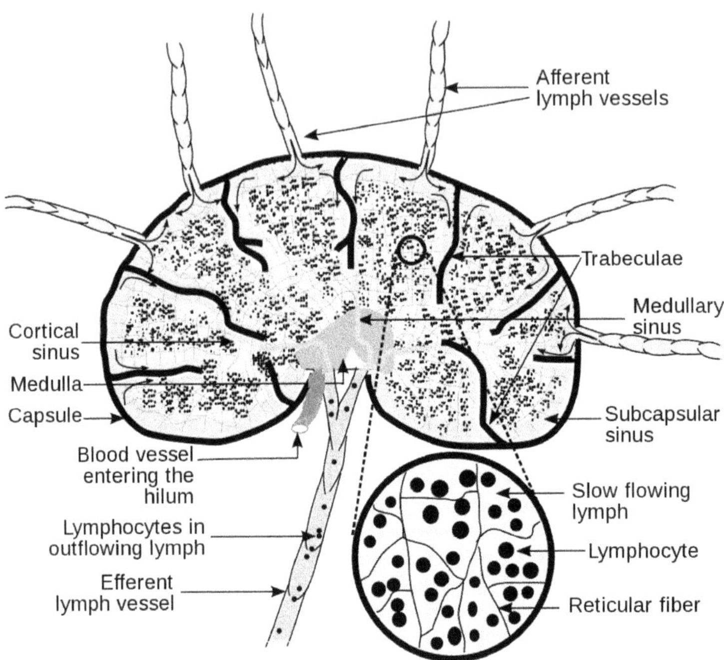

IMG: LYMPH NODE _IMG CREDIT KC PANCHAL

Lymph node

- lymph node possess a fibrous tissue capsule
- it consists of an outer cortex and inner medulla
- cortex contains lymphoid follicles with germinal centres
- paracortex is the junction between cortex and medulla, it contains T-lymphocytes
- Medulla contains medullary cords and sinusoidS

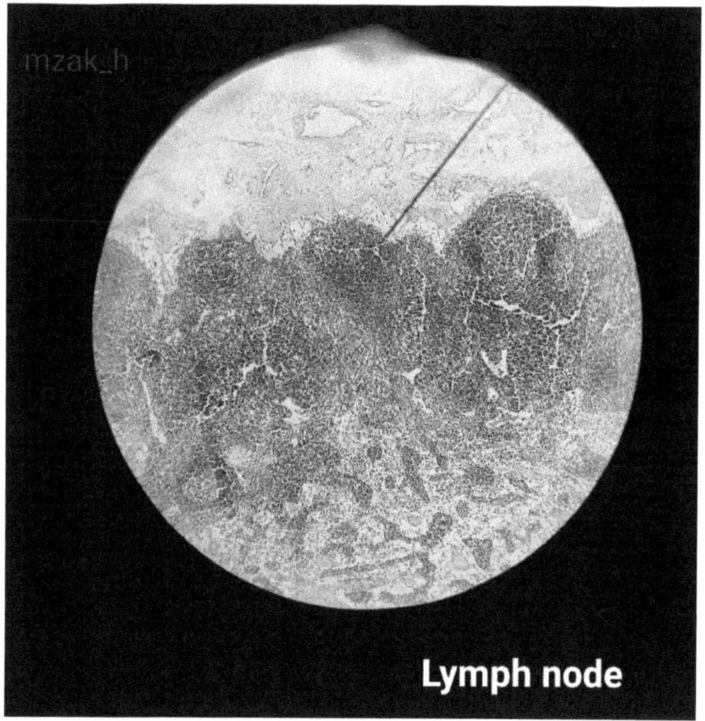

LYMPH NODE

Spleen

- possess a fibrous capsule
- it is shows red and white pulp

White pulp

- consist of lymphoid aggregations with eccentric Central artery

Red pulp

- contains RBC, macrophages, Lymphocytes and monocytes

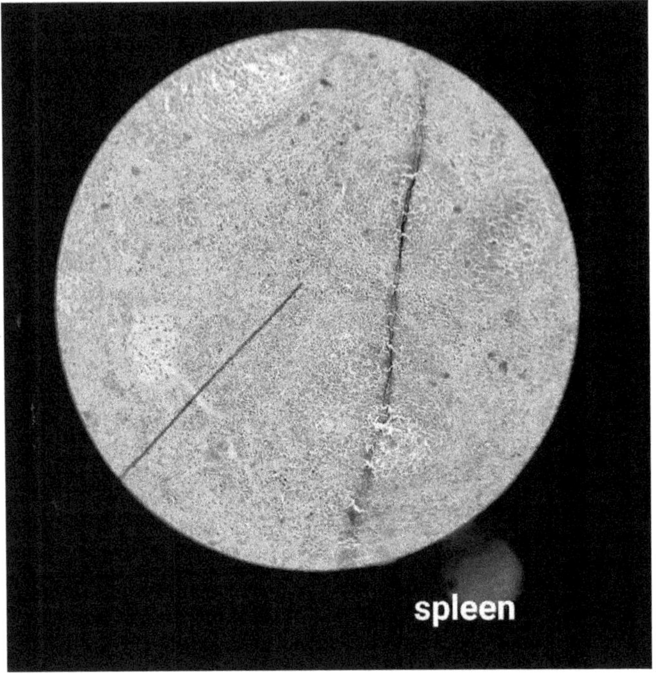

SPLEEN

Tonsil

- tonsillar crypts are present
- lined by stratified squamous non keratinized epithelium
- lymphoid follicles with the germinal centres are seen along the crypts
- germinalcentres are seen along the crypts

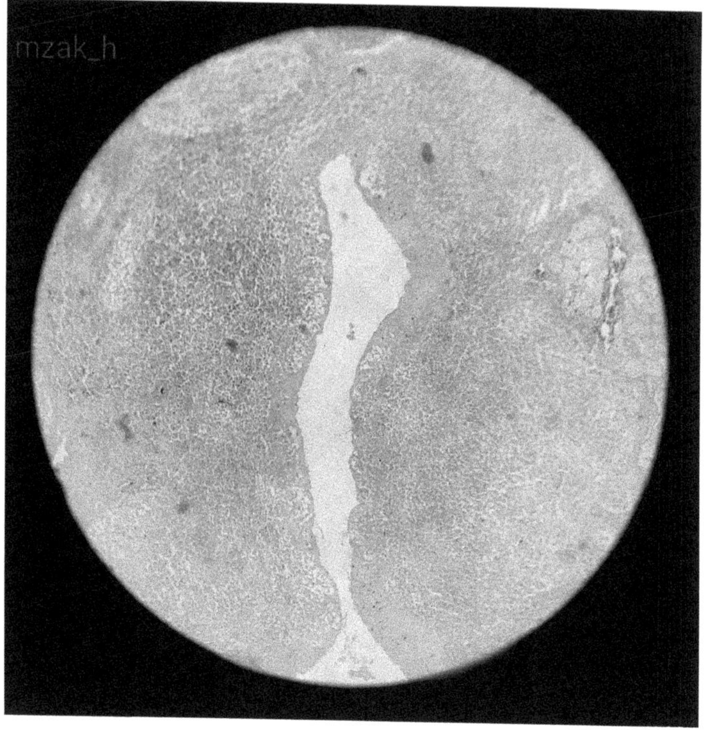

TONSIL

Thymus

- Septa incompletely divides the lobes into irregular lobules
- Each lobule possess outer cortex and inner medulla
- outer cortex is darkly stained and consisting of lymphocytes
- Inner medulla is lightly stained and possess hassall's corpuscles

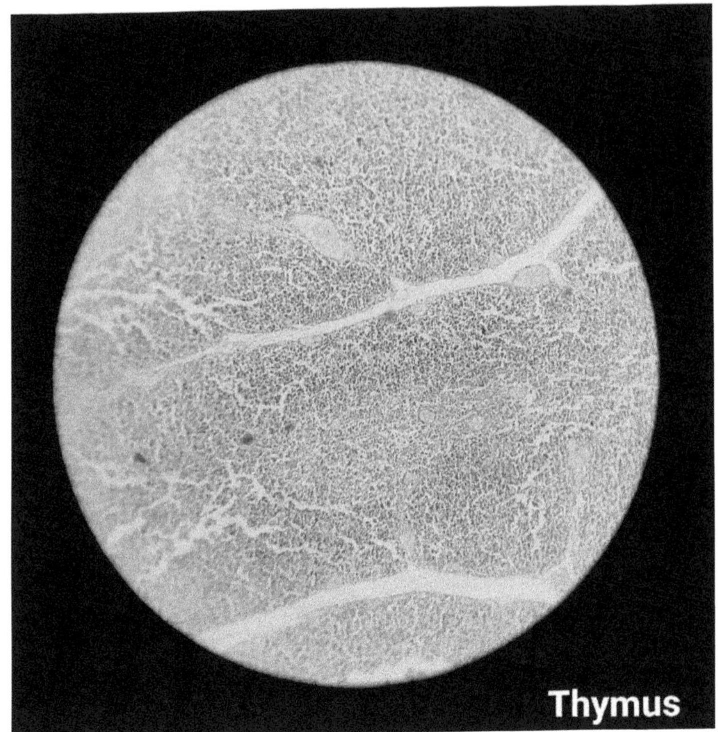
Thymus

• • •

CHAPTER XI

GALLBLADDER

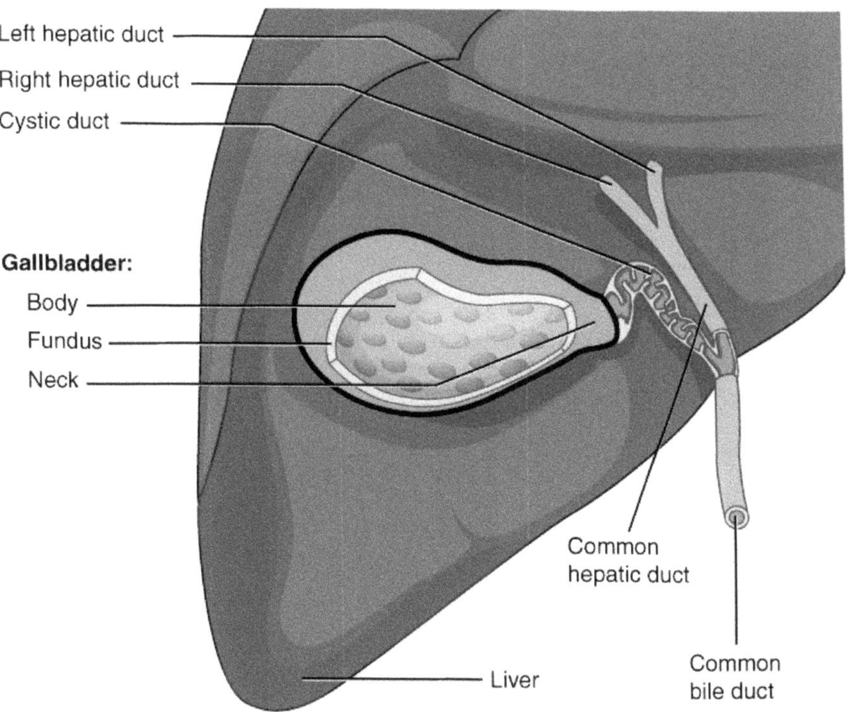

img: gallbladder (img credit:By OpenStax College - Anatomy & Physiology, Connexions Web site. http://cnx.org/content/col11496/1.6/, Jun 19, 2013., CC BY 3.0, https://commons.wikimedia.org/w/index.php?curid=30148460)

Gallbladder is a muscular sac It consists of 3 layers

Mucosa

- Lined by simple tall columnar epithelium.
- The columnar epithelium possess microvilli for absorption of water.
- Lamina propria of mucosa is rich in elastic fibres.
- When bladder is empty, mucosa is thrown into small folds.

[*Muscularis mucosa & submucosa absent*]

Fibromuscular layer

- Made up of connective tissues and smooth muscle fibres.

Serosa / Adventitia

- made up of connective tissue

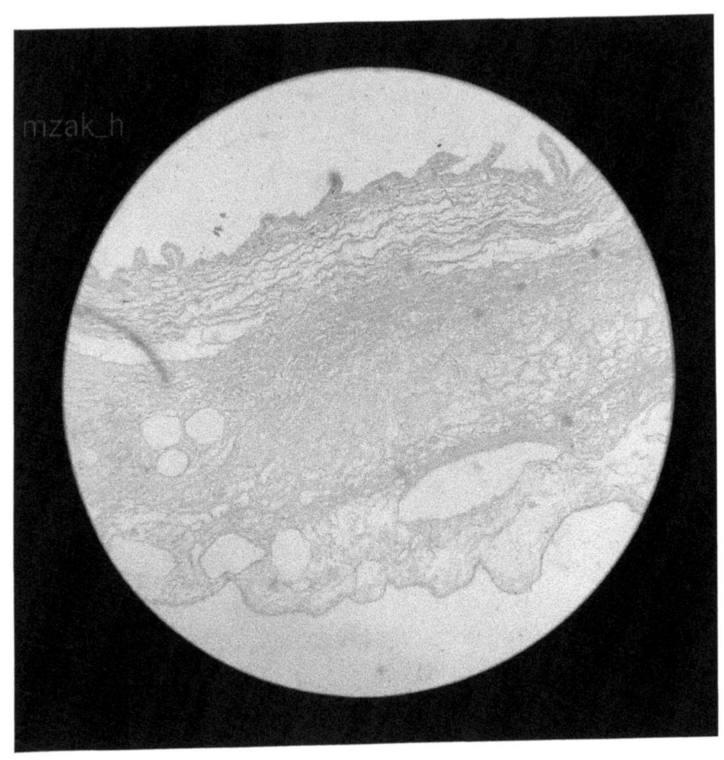

H&E SLIDE GALLBLADDER

• • •

CHAPTER XII

TONGUE

in tongue we can observe 3 types of papillae

1. Filiform
2. fungiform
3. circumvallate

filiform papillae are lined by" keratinized stratified squamous epithelium" and others are lined by" non keratinized stratified squamous epithelium"

all papillae except filiform papillae, shows taste buds

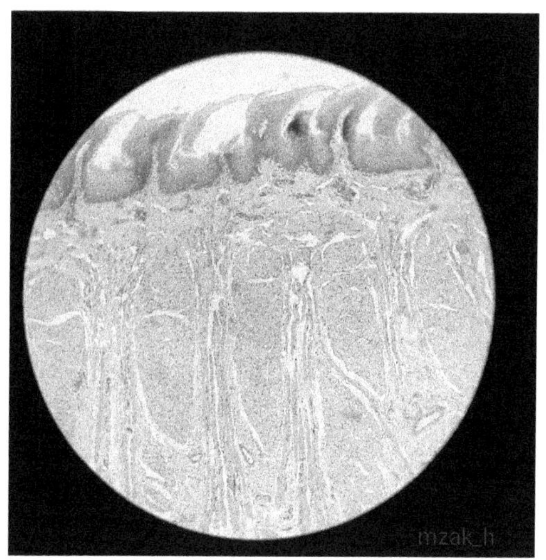

TONGUE

• • •

CHAPTER XIII

SKIN

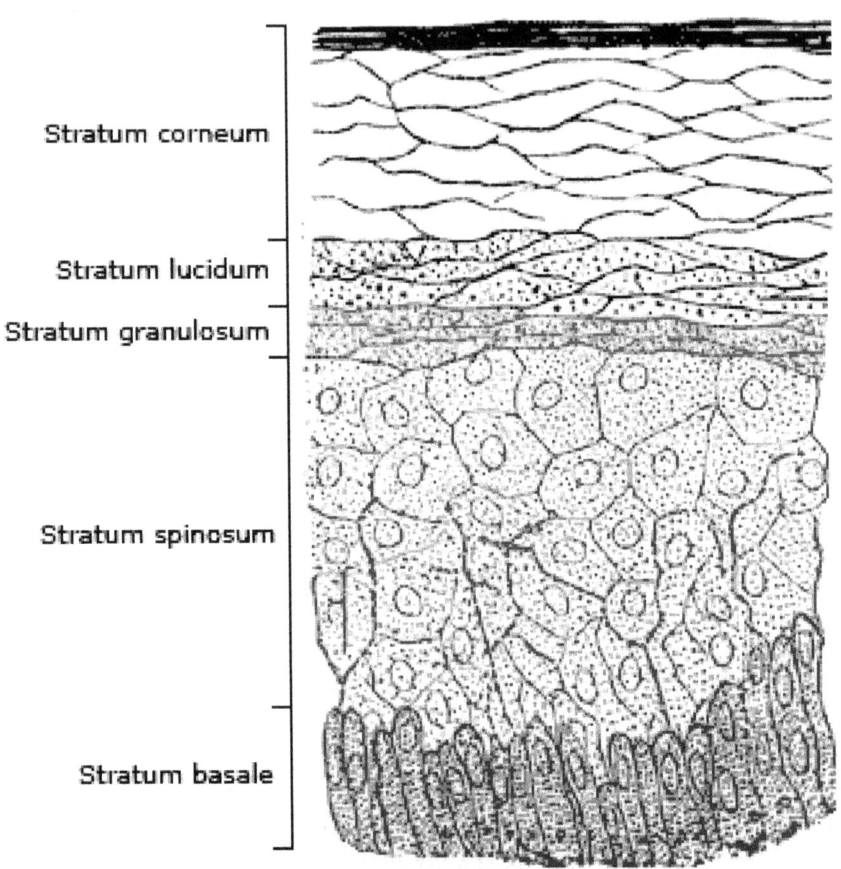

LAYERS OF EPIDERMIS_ IMAGE CREDIT: Modified from the original Grey's diagram here

skin is made up of three layers :

1. Epidermis
2. Dermis

3. Subcutaneous layer(hypodermis)

- epidermis has following layers(from deep to superficial)

Stratum basale

This is the deepest layer consisting of cuboidal or columnar cells. They show mitotic activity. They undergo mitosis and give rise to new melanocytes

Stratum spinosum

Composed of polyhedral cells held together by Desmosomes

Stratum granulosum

made up of three to five layers of flattened, fusiform cells. They are filled with keratohyalin granules

Stratum lucidum

It is made up of flattened, eosinophilic, dead cells. Cytoplasm of these cells are filled with keratin. This layer has a classy appearance

Stratum corneum

it is the most superficial layer consists of non- -nucleated, dead, scaly and keratinized

Thick skin

- Thick epidermis (stratum corneum is thick)
- Hair follicles and sebaceous glands are absent
- sweat glands are present in epidermis

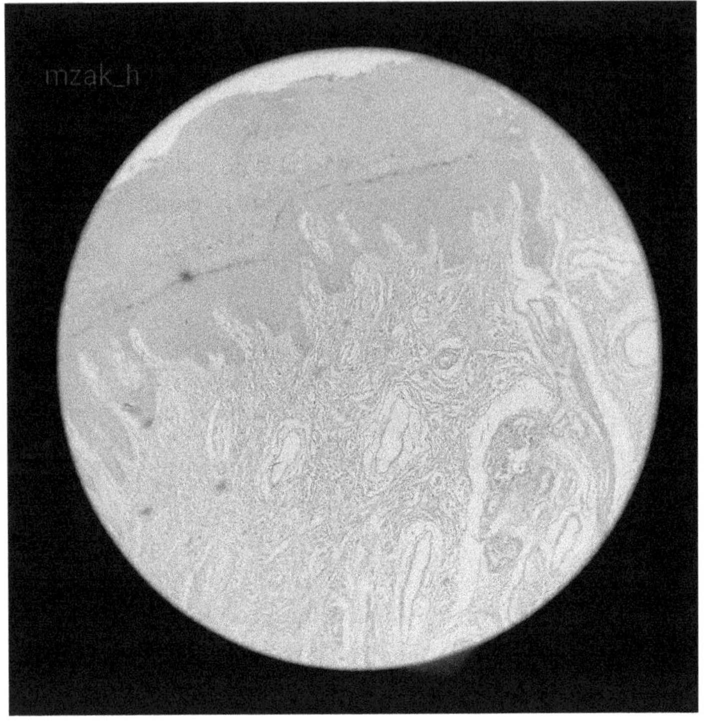

THICK SKIN

Thin skin

- Thin epidermis (stratum corneum is thin)
- Hair follicles and sebaceous glands are present
- Sweat glands are present in dermis

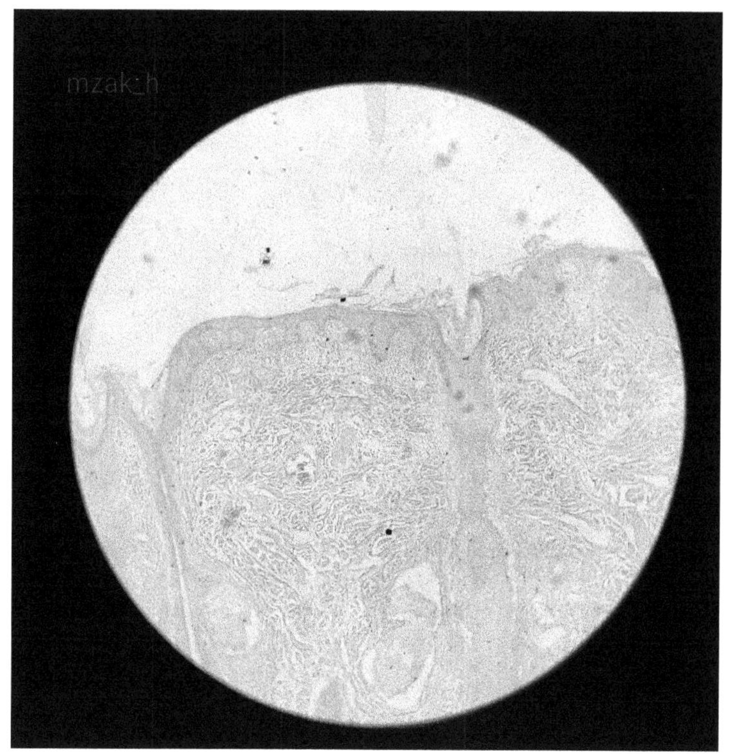

THIN SKIN

• • •

CHAPTER XIV

TRACHEA AND LUNG

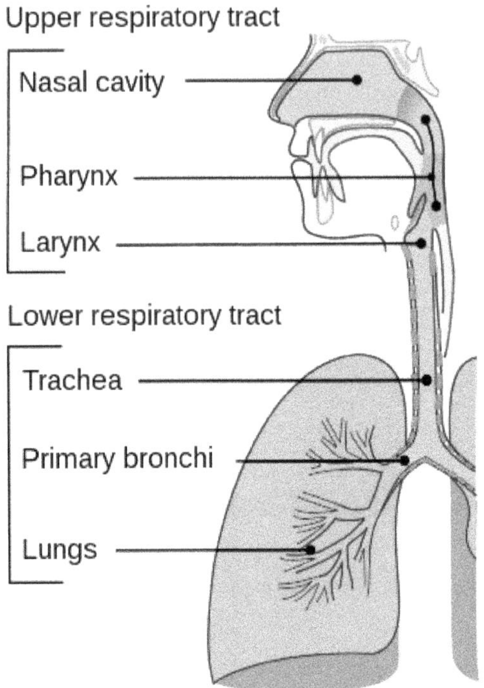

IMG: HUMAN RESPIRATORY SYSTEM

TRACHEA

has following parts:

- MUCOSA
- SUBMUCOSA

- CARTILAGE AND MUSCLE LAYER
- ADVENTIA

1.MUCOSA

lined by "pseudostratified ciliated columnar epithelium" with goblet cells(aka respiratory epithelium)

2.SUBMUCOSA

submucosa is composed of loose connective tissue.It contains blood vessels,nerves,lymphatics and lot of serous and mucous glands

3.CARTILLAGE AND MUSCLE LAYER

Consists of C-shaped hyaline cartilage with perichondrium.Posterior ends of cartilages are connected together by"trachealis muscle".

4.ADVENTIA

made up of connective tissue with blood vessels

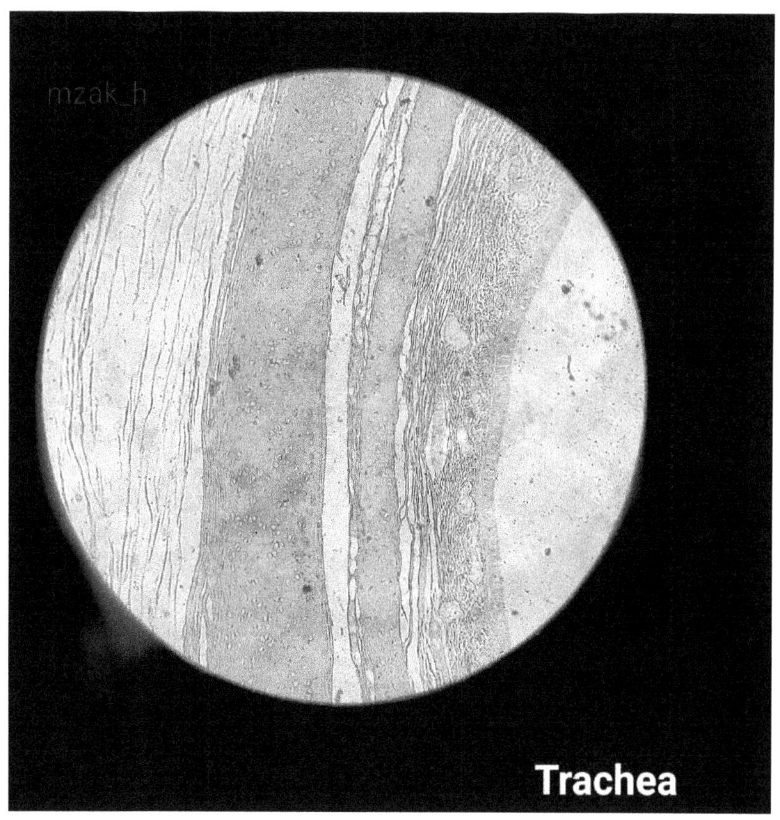

LUNG

- Secondary and tertiary bronchi are lined by pseudostratified ciliated columnar epithelium with few goblet cells
- Bronchioles: simple columnar or cuboidal ciliated epithelium with no Goblet cells
- Terminal bronchioles: Simple columnar
- Respiratory bronchioles: Cuboidal epithelium
- Alveoli: Squamous epithelium

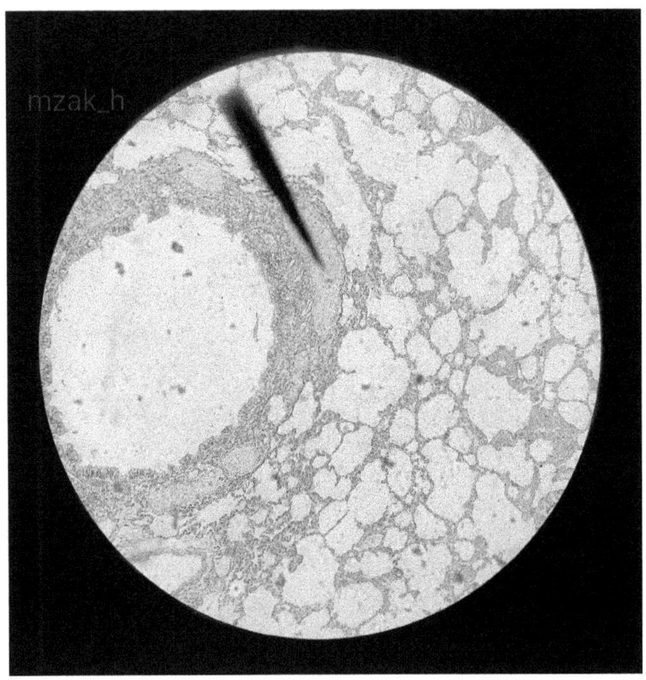

LUNG

• • •

CHAPTER XV

CARTILAGE

Cartilage is a special dense connective tissue.

Cells of cartilage are:-

- Chondrocytes (mature)
- Chondroblast (immature)

Intracellular matrix of cartilage consists of:

- Fibers- type I/ type II collagen & elastic fibers
- Ground substances- made up of glycoproteins (so stains basic)

Note: All the cartilages are covered by perichondrium

- Outer fibrous
- Inner cellular type

HYALINE CARTILAGE

➡Characterized by "Translucent homogenous bluish matrix"

- Translucent – because the presence of proteoglycans in matrix
- Bluish matrix – due to the presence of proteoglycan, matrix is basophilic so it is stained by hematoxylin
- Homogeneous – because the refractive index of collagen fibers and ground substance is same

➡Here chondrocytes lie within the lacunae and they are arranged in groups of 2- 6 cells called "cell nest"

➡ Matrix around the cell nest we can observe lightly stained interterritorial matrix

➡Examples: articular cartilage, epiphyseal plate, costal cartilage.

Note:

- collagen fibers present in hyaline cartilage are type II
- Articular cartilage is devoid of perichondrium
- H&E slide low magnification view hyaline cartilage

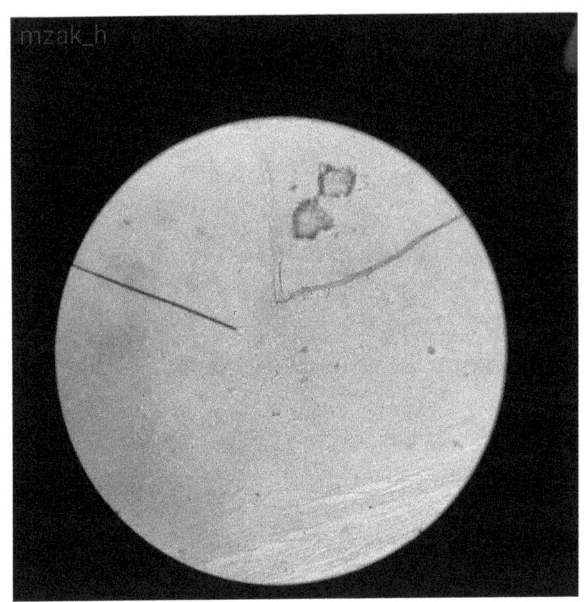

HYALINE CARTILAGE

ELASTIC CARTILAGE

- Perichondrium present
- Chondrocytes are larger than those of hyaline cartilage and are present "singly"or in small groups (groups of two or three)
- Matrix is eosinophilic (stained by eosin) with abundance of anastomosing elastic fibres
- Show elasticity
- Examples- epiglottis, eustachian tube,external acoustic meatus,pinna,parts of corniculate and cuneiform cartilage of larynx

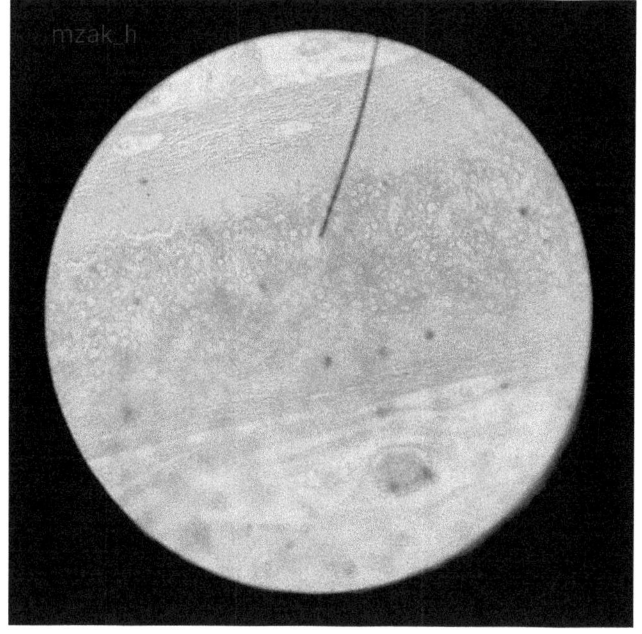

ELASTIC CARTILAGE

FIBROUS CARTILAGE

- chondrocytes are small and very few in number
- chondrocytes are arranged in rows in b/w bundles of type I collagen fibres
- Examples :Intervertebral disc, cartilage of Pubic symphysis, menisci of knee joint,articular disc of TM joint and sternoclavicular joint.

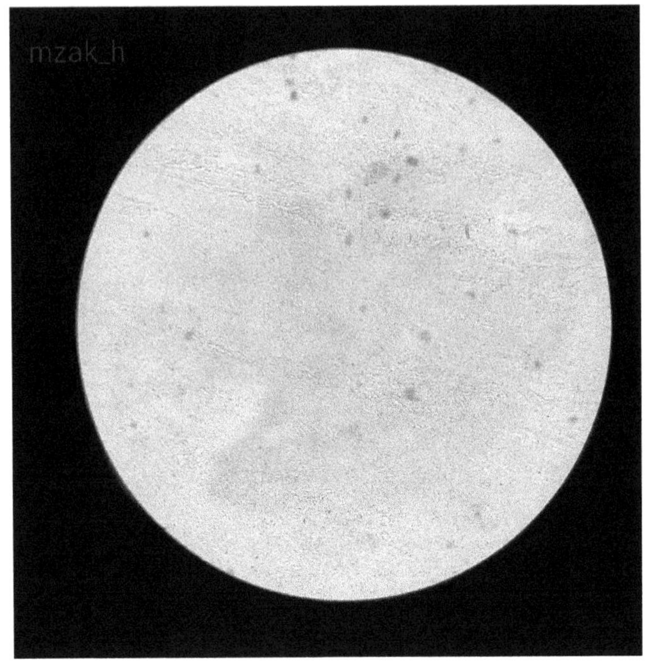

FIBROUS CARTILAGE

• • •

CHAPTER XVI

URINARY SYSTEM

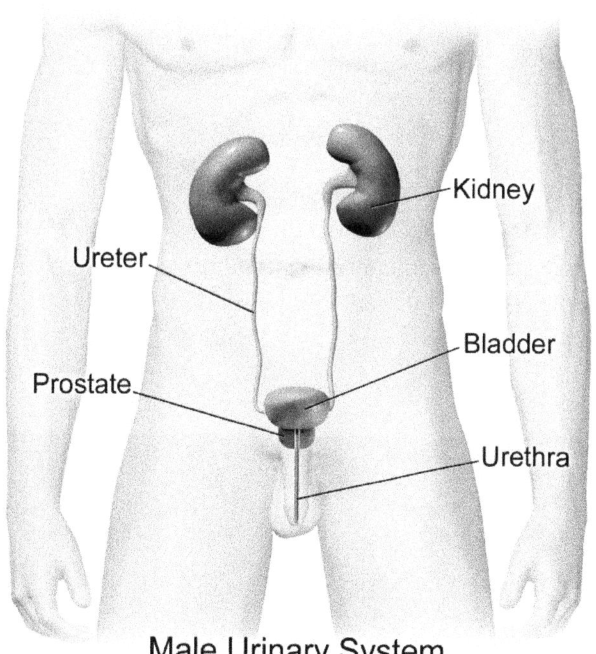

(img credit: By BruceBlaus - Own work, CC BY-SA 4.0, https://commons.wikimedia.org/w/index.php?curid=61465355)

Kidney

- kidney consists of outer cortex and inner medulla

Cortex

consist of

1. Renal corpuscles
2. pct- lined with cuboidal cells with microvilli
3. dct- lined with squamous to cuboidal cells

Medulla

consist of

1. collecting tubule-cuboidal epithelium
2. collecting ducts-cuboidal epithelium
3. loop of henle (thick) - squamous epithelium
4. loop of henle (thin) - cuboidal epithelium
5. vasa recta-endothelium

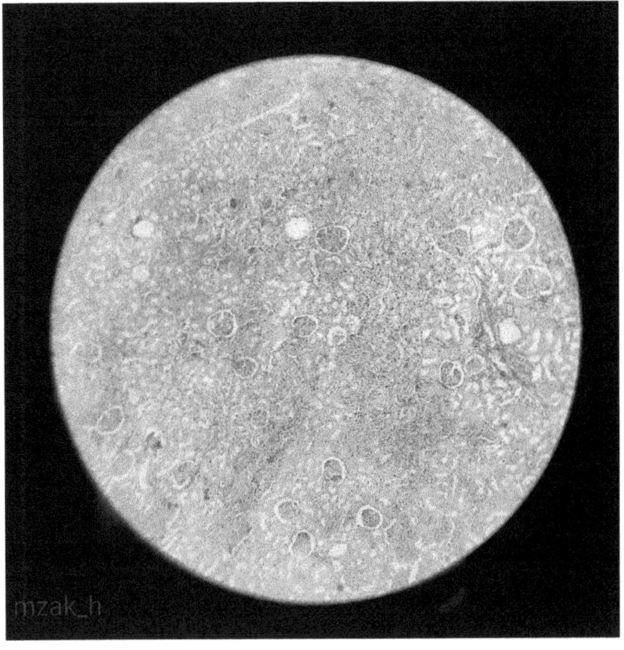

H&E SLIDE KIDNEY

Ureter

Mucosa

- shows longitudinal folds, lined by transitional epithelium
- lamina propria consists of connective tissue

Muscular coat

- inner circular and Outer longitudinal

Adventitia

- made up of connective tissue

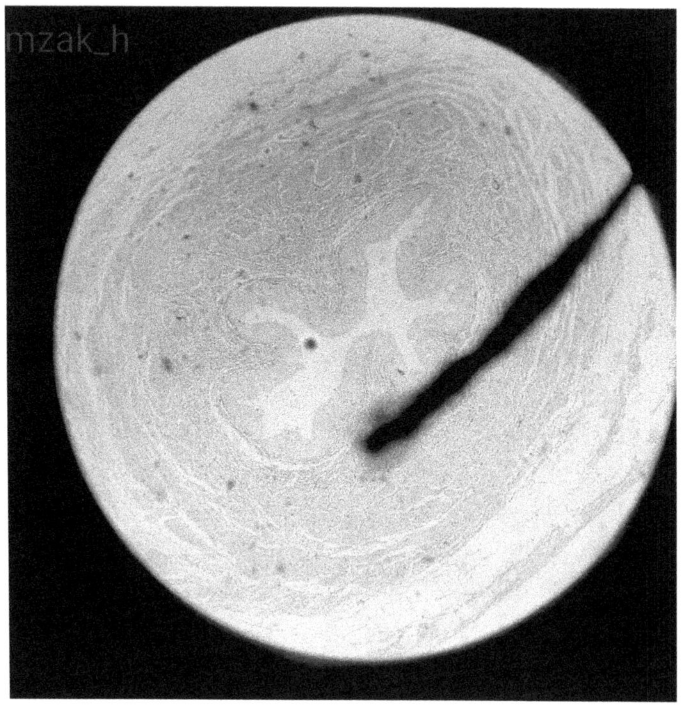

H&E SLIDE URETER

Urinary bladder

Mucosa

- consists of transitional epithelial lining and lamina propria

Muscle coat

- Thick muscle coat with ill-defined layers

Adventitia

- made of connective tissue

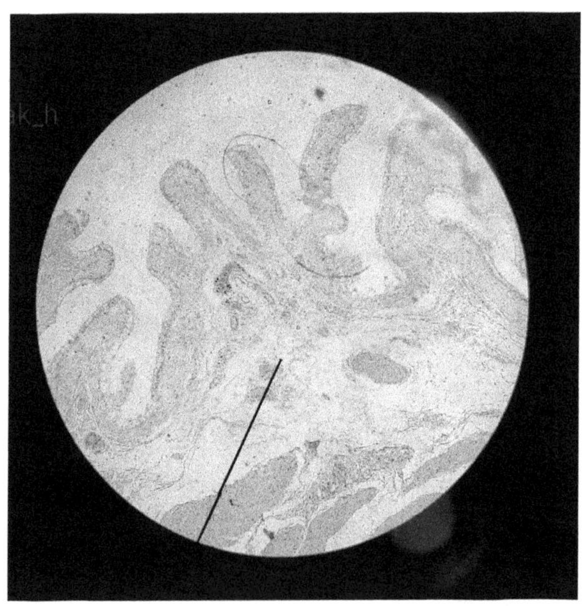

H&E SLIDE URINARY BLADDER

• • •

CHAPTER XVII

ADRENAL, PITUTARY & THYROID

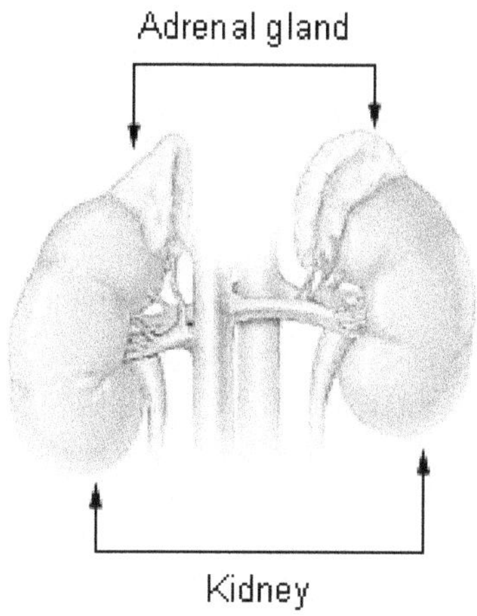

IMG:ADRENAL GLAND (IMG CREDIT-EEOC - cancer.gov)

ADRENAL GLAND

Consist of adrenal cortex and adrenal medulla

Adrenal cortex

- Consist of 3 zones

1. Zona glomerulosa- consists of short Columnar cells, which are Arranged as "curved-columns"
2. Zona fasciculata-consist of polyhedral cells which are arranged as linear columns
3. Zona reticularis - arranged as cell networks

Adrenal medulla

- consists of chromaffin cells which are arranged in between sinusoids

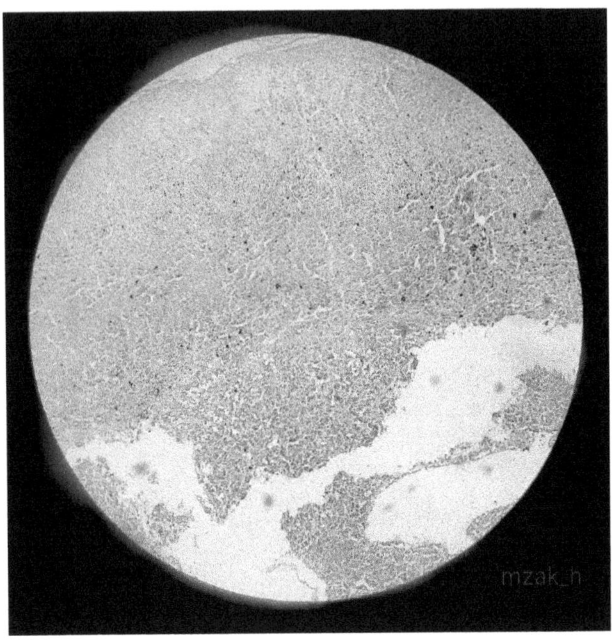

ADRENAL GLAND

Thyroid gland

- thyroid follicles are lined with simple cuboidal epithelium
- thyroid follicles are filled with colloid or thyroglobulin
- parafollicular cells are seen between thyroid follicles

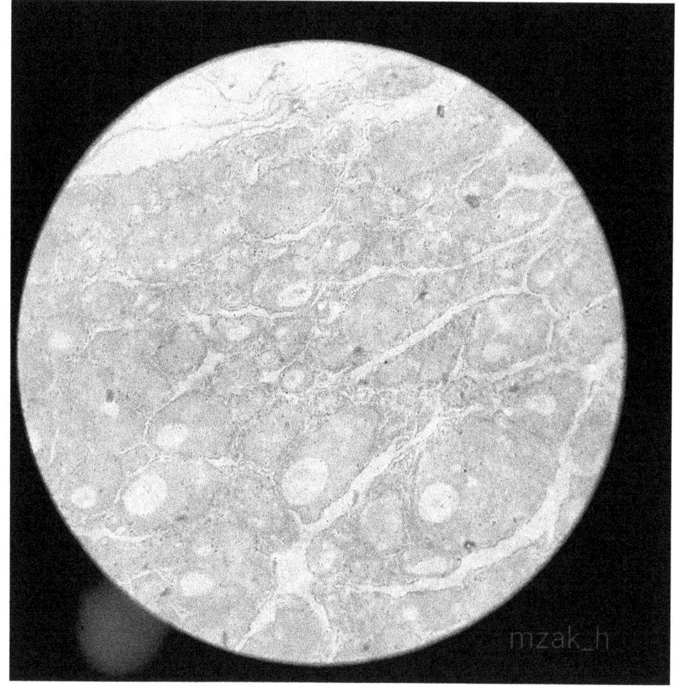

THYROID GLAND

Pituitary

Pituitary gland has 3 lobes

1. anterior lobe(pars anterior)
2. intermediate lobe(pars intermedia)
3. posterior lobe

Anterior lobe

Consist of three types of cells

1)acidophils-consist of somatotrophs and Lactotrophs

2)basophils-consist of gonadotropes,Thyrotropes & Corticotrophs

3)chromophoes-No hormonal function

Posterior lobe

Consist of large number of nerve fibers

Intermediate lobe

Contains large number of pale cells which usually surround follicles, filled with colloids

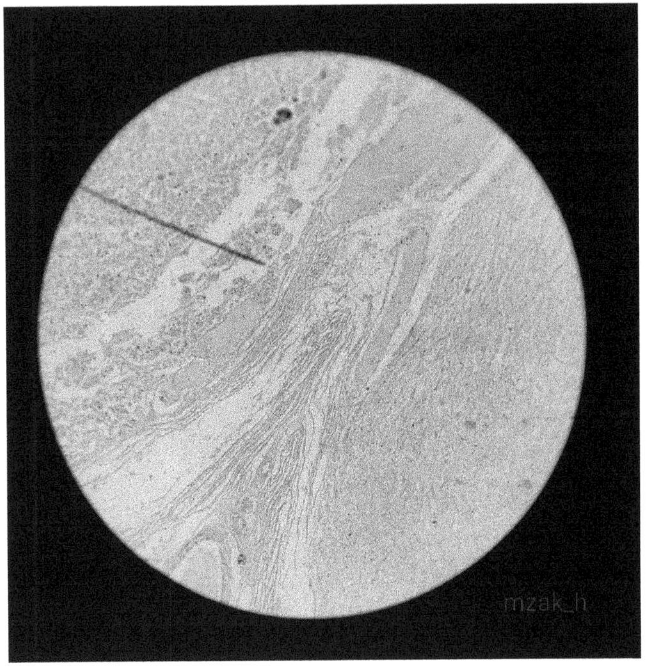

PITUTARY

• • •

CHAPTER XVIII

NERVOUS SYSTEM

CEREBELLUM

Consist of folia with outer cortex and inner medulla

Cerebellar cortex consists of 3 layers

1. Molecular layer- consist of stellate and Basket cells
2. Purkinje cell layer - Purkinje cells
3. Granule cell layer- granular cells and golgi cells

Cerebellar medulla consists of white matter fibers

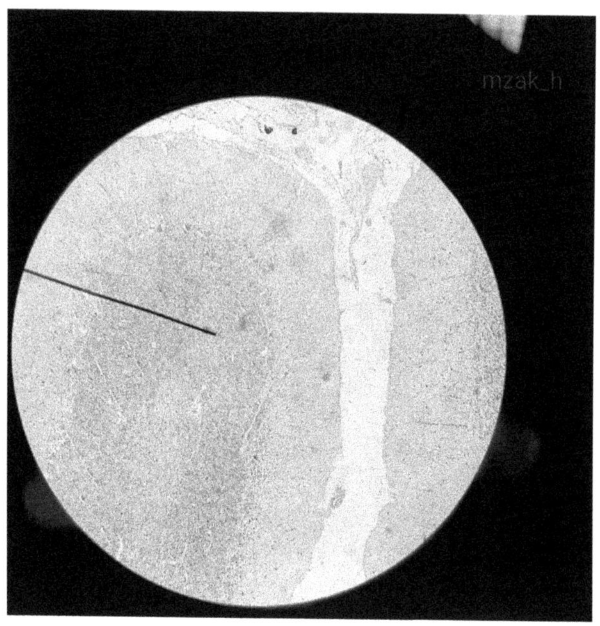

H&E SLIDE CEREBELLUM

CEREBRUM

cerebrum consist of 6 layers

1. Molecular layer consists of mainly nerve fibres and occasionally horizontal cells of cajal
2. Outer granular layer consists of stellate and small pyramidal cells
3. Pyramidal layer consists of medium sized pyramidal cells,stellate cells and cells of martinotti
4. Inner granular layer consist of stellate cells
5. Ganglionic layer consists of large pyramidal cells and few stellate cells
6. Polymorphous layer consists of nerve fibres, stellate cells and the cells of martinotti

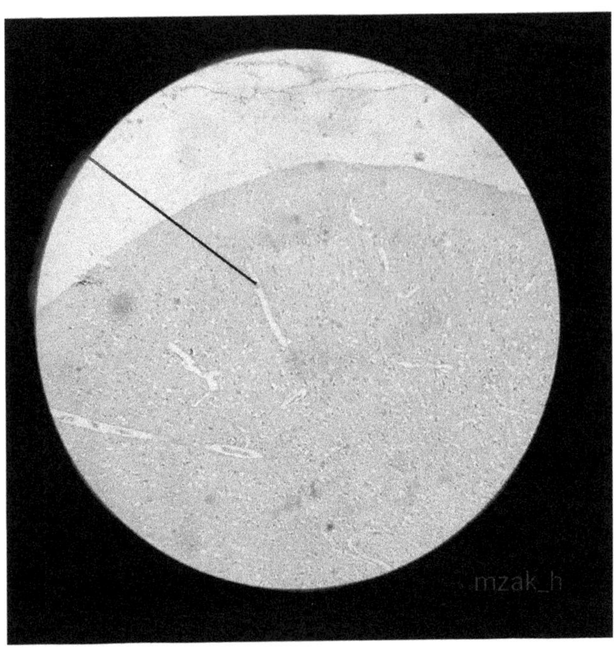

H&E SLIDE CREBRUM

Spinal cord

- consist of Central"H "shaped grey matter with the large anterior horns and narrow posterior horns
- possess a central canal

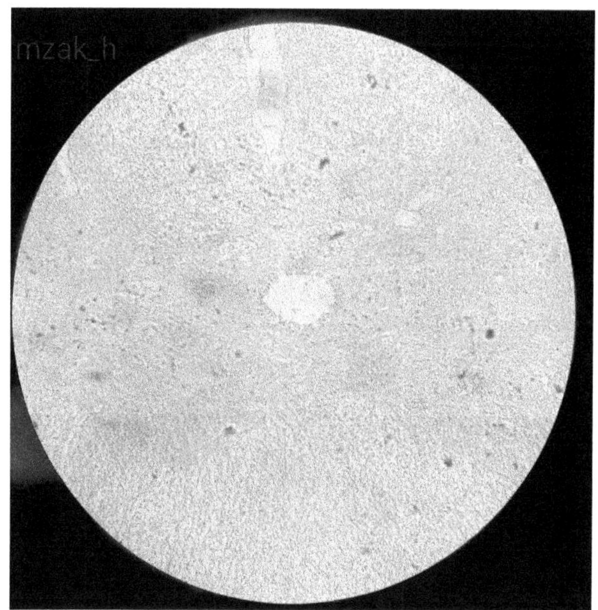

H&E SLIDE SPINAL CORD

CHAPTER XIX

MAMMARY GLAND

Inactive mammary gland

- more connective tissue, less glandular tissue
- underdeveloped alveoli with small lumen
- extensive branching of ducts

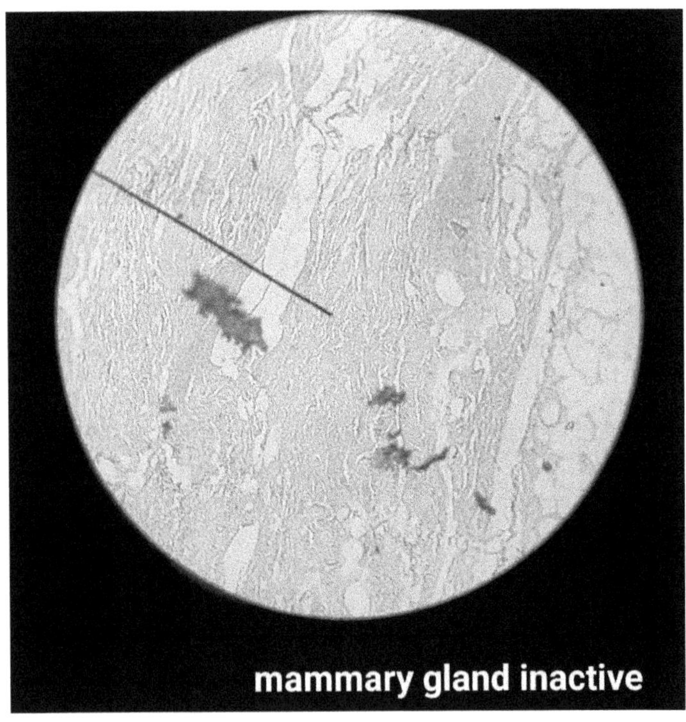

MAMMARY GLAND INACTIVE

Active mammary glands

- less connective tissue and more glandular tissue
- compactly packed, well developed alveoli with distended lumen containing milk

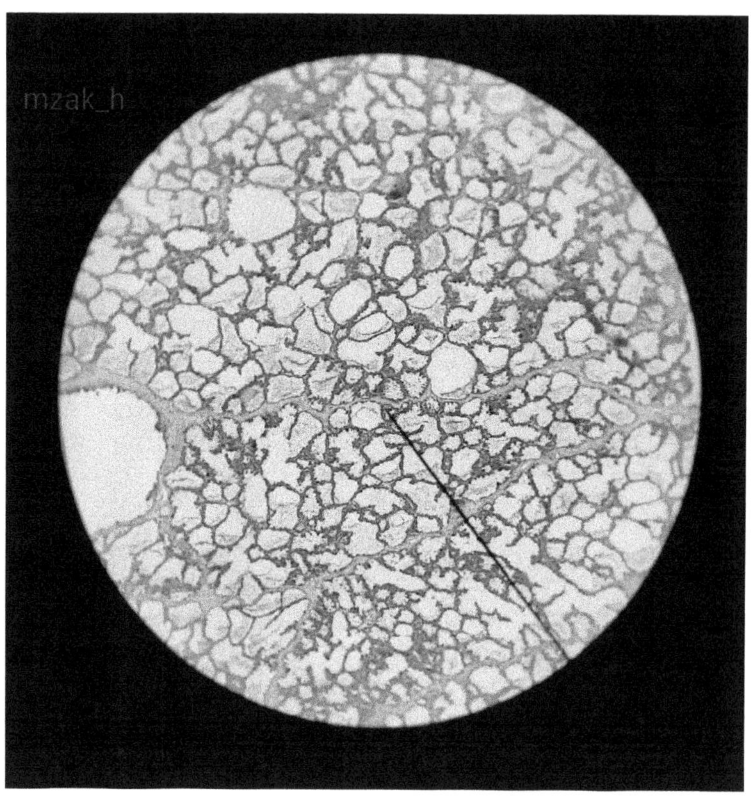

MAMMARY GLAND ACTIVE

CHAPTER XX

OVARY

Covering of ovary : outer germinal epithelium and inner tunica albuginea

- Parts of ovary parts of ovary are outer cortex and inner medulla
- cortex shows ovarian follicles in different stages of development
- medulla consists of connective tissues and blood vessels

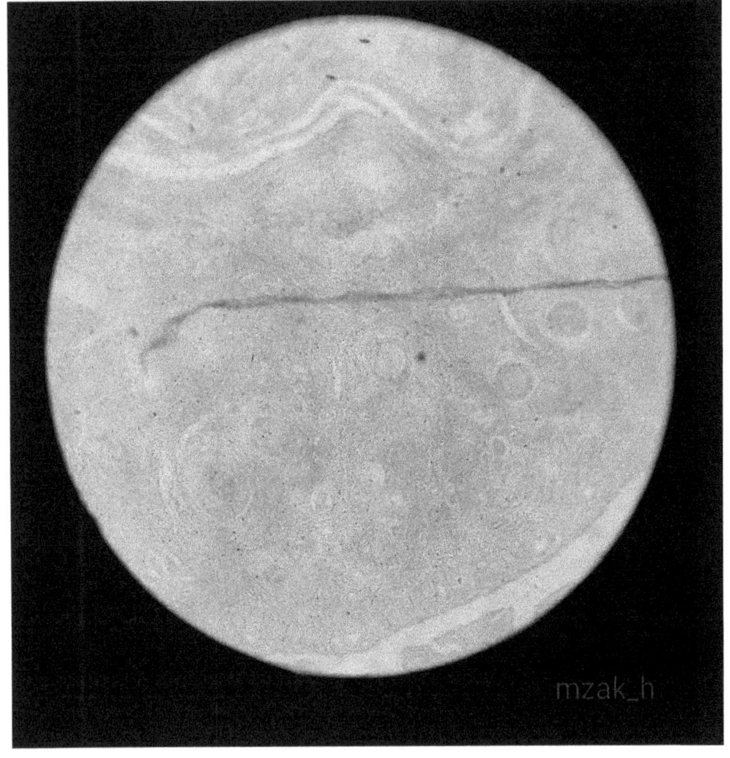

H&E SLIDE OVARY

• • •

CHAPTER XXI

UTERUS

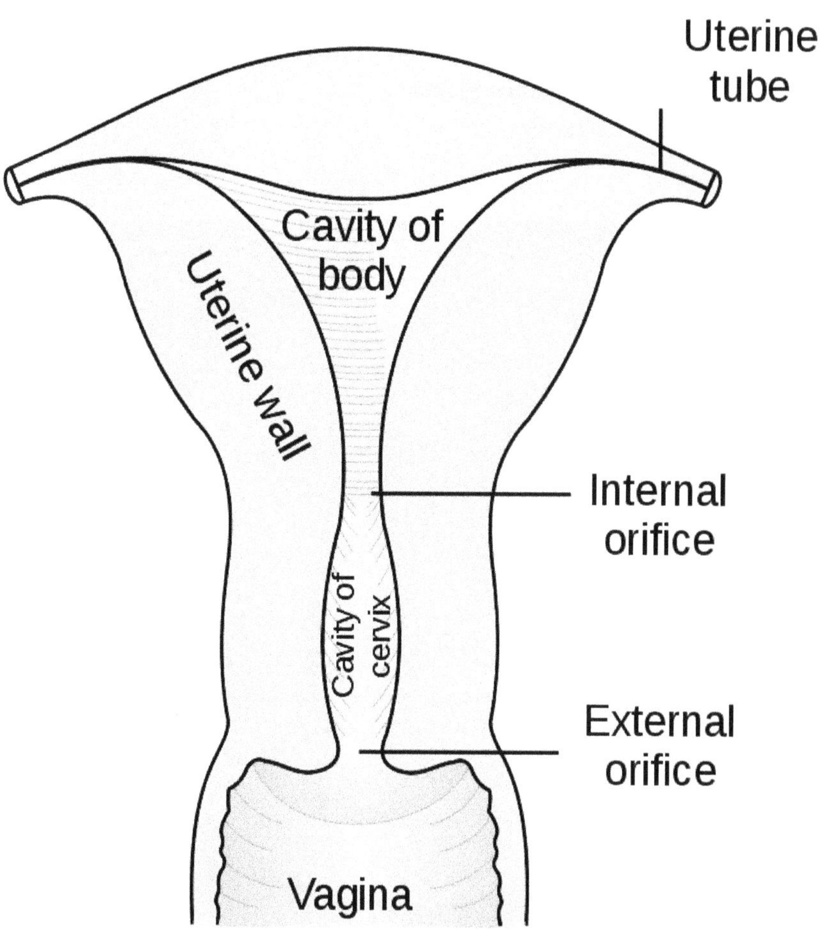

IMG: UTERUS (IMAGE CREDIT: HENDRY GRAY)

Uterus has three layers endometrium, myometrium & perimetrium

Endometrium

CHAPTER XXII

FALLOPIAN TUBE

Mucosa

- consist of lining epithelium and lamina propria
- mucosa is highly folded and lined by ciliated columnar epithelium

Muscle layer

- inner circular and Outer longitudinal smooth muscle layers

Serosa-mesothelium

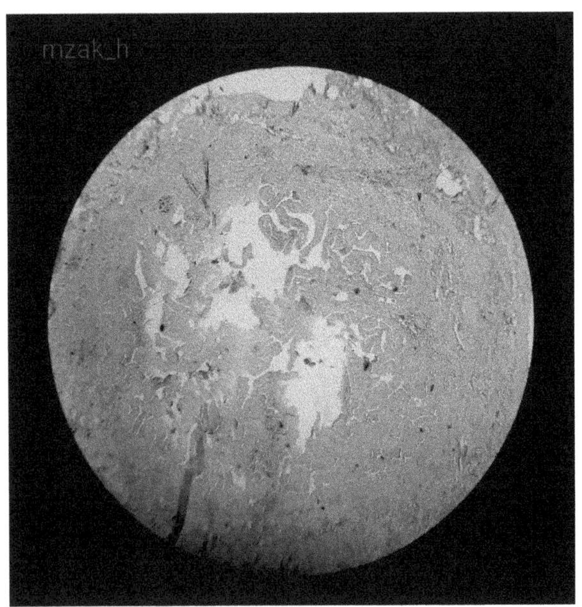

H&E SLIDE FALLOPIAN TUBE

• • •

CHAPTER XXIII

MALE REPRODUCTIVE SYSTEM

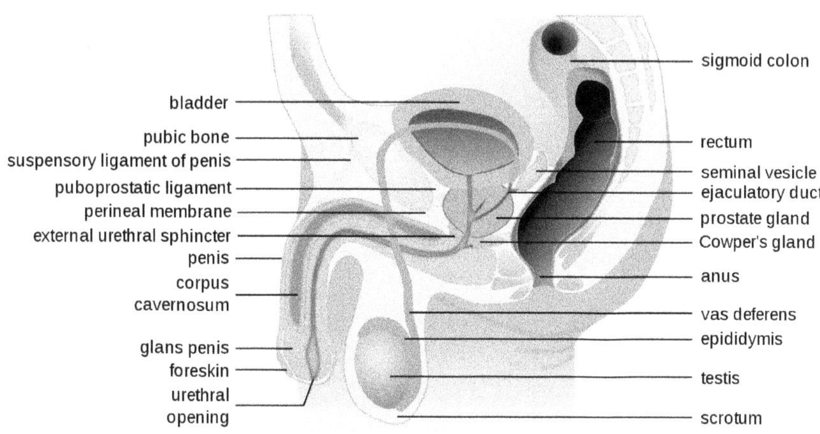

(img credit; By Male_anatomy.png: alt.sex FAQderivative work: Tsaitgaist (talk) - *[[:File:Male_anatomy.png|Male_anatomy.png], CC BY-SA 3.0, https://commons.wikimedia.org/w/index.php?curid=6569849)

Prostate

histologically prostate consists of parenchyma and fibromuscular stroma

Glandular parenchyma

- formed by irregular prostatic alveoli
- lined by cuboidal to columnar epithelium depending upon activity
- Amyloid bodies(colloid) found in the lumen of alveoli

Stroma

- consist of fibrous tissue and smooth muscles

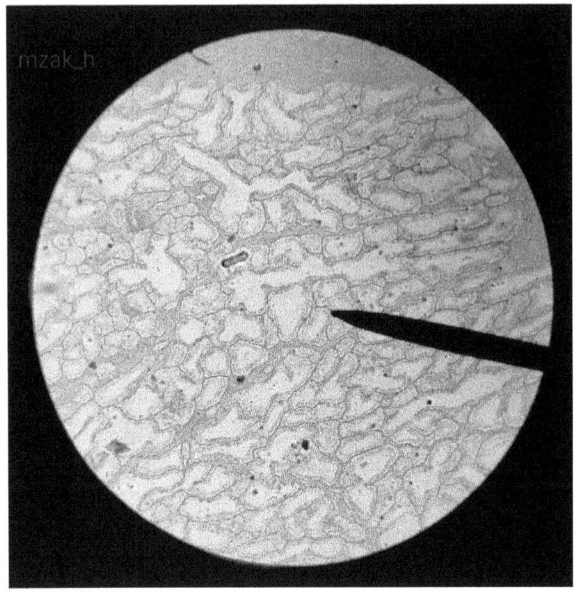

H&E SLIDE PROSTATE

Vas deferens

Consist of

MUCOSA

- consist of simple or pseudostratified columnar epithelial lining and underlying lamina propria

MUSCLE COAT

- thick, large, muscle coat consists of inner longitudinal, middle circular & outer longitudinal smooth muscles

ADVENTITIA

- made up of connective tissue

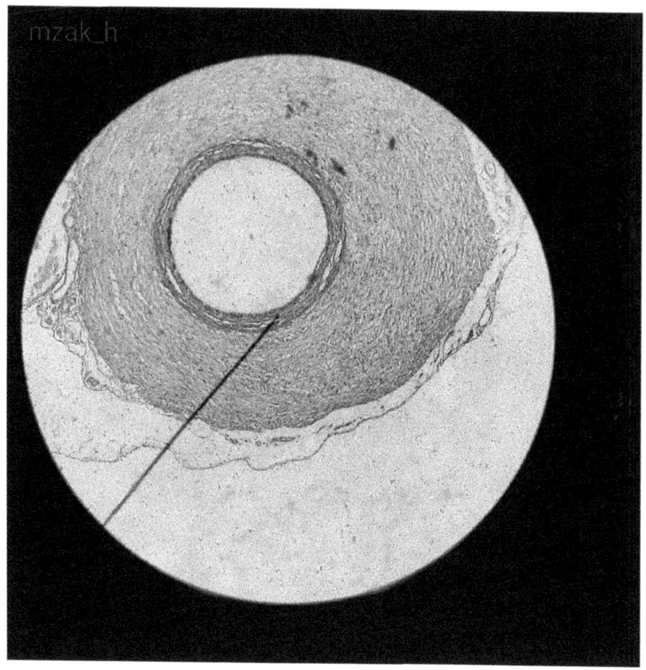

vas deferens

Testis

Characterized by seminiferous tubules, lined with:-

1)spermatogonia

2)different stages of spermatocytes

3)sertoli cells

Sertoli cells are tall columnar cells with prominent nucleus

In between seminiferous tubules we can observe androgen secreting" leydig cells"

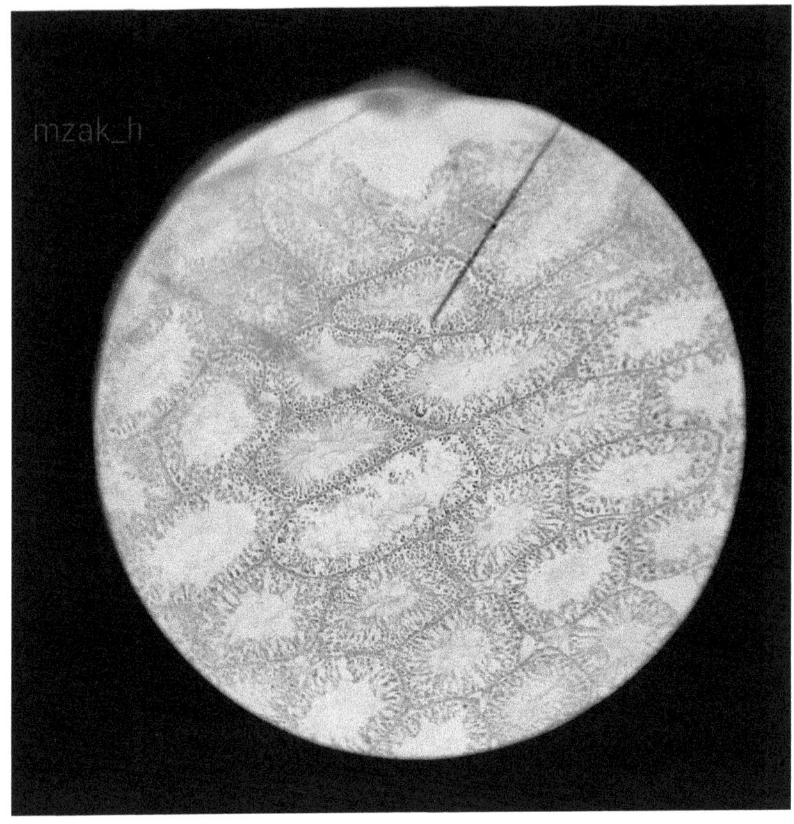

H&E SLIDE TESTIS

Epididymis

- epididymis is a comma shaped structure on the posterior- lateral aspect of testis
- it is composed of 6cm long tubes, called "ductus epididymis "which are supported by connective tissue
- ductus epididymis is lined by pseudostratified columnar epithelium with stereocilia
- smooth muscle fibres surrounding each ductus
- Sperms are in the lumen

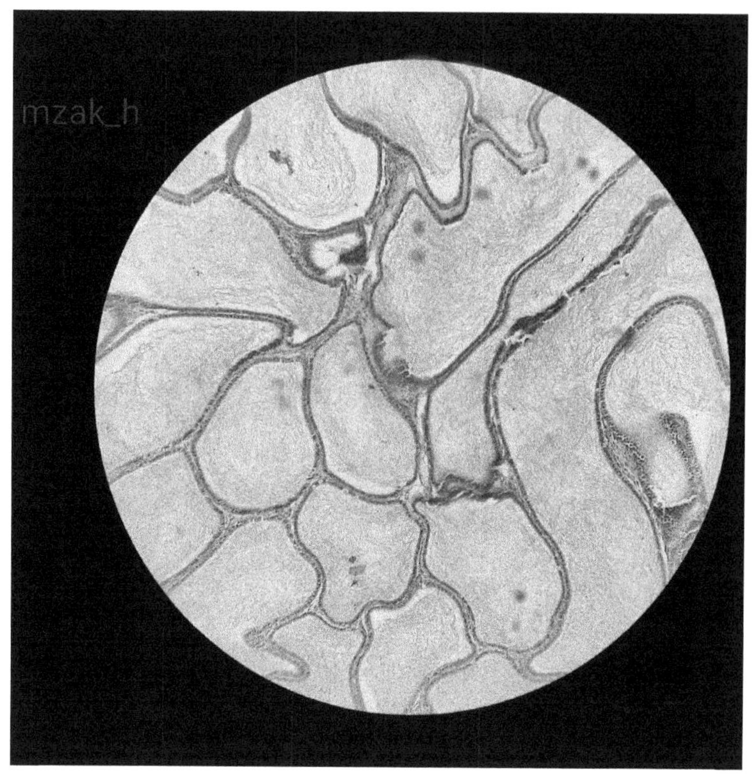

H&E SLIDE EPIDIDYMIS

• • •

CHAPTER XXIV

EYE

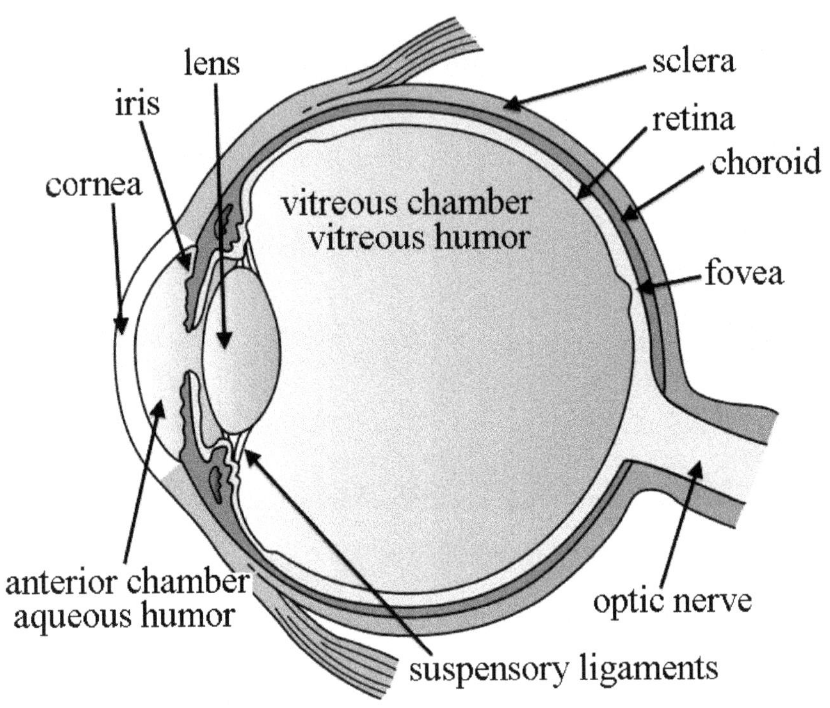

IMAGE EYE_ (IMG CREDIT:By Artwork by Holly Fischer - http://open.umich.edu/education/med/resources/second-look-series/materials - Eye Slide 3, CC BY 3.0, https://commons.wikimedia.org/w/index.php?curid=24367145)

Cornea

Consist of

1. Corneal epithelium stratified squamous non keratinized epithelium
2. Bowman's membrane it is the basement membrane of corneal epithelium
3. Substantia propria composed of parallel bundles of collagen and corneal cells
4. Descemet's membrane also known as posterior limiting membrane
5. Posterior epithelium (endothelium)

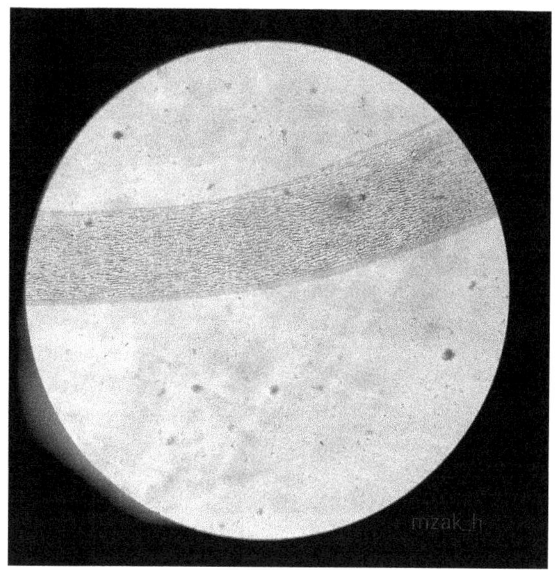

H&E SLIDE CORNEA

Retina

Consist of 10 layers

1. pigment epithelium
2. layers of rods and cones
3. outer limiting membrane
4. outer nuclear layer
5. outer plexiform layer
6. inner nuclear layer

7. inner plexiform layer
8. ganglion cell layer
9. nuclear fibre layer
10. inner limiting membrane

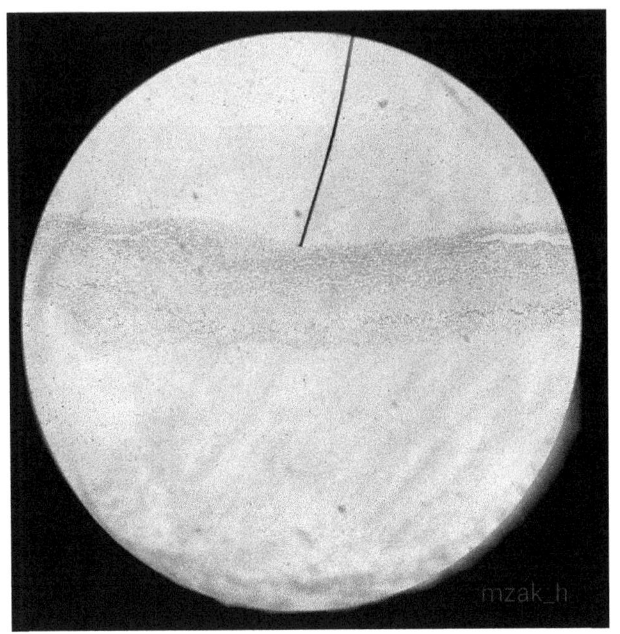

H&E SLIDE RETINA

• • •

CHAPTER XXV

EMBRYOLOGICAL TISSUE

Placenta

- Maternal part-decidua basalis
- Fetal part-chorion frondosum which give rise to Chorionic villi

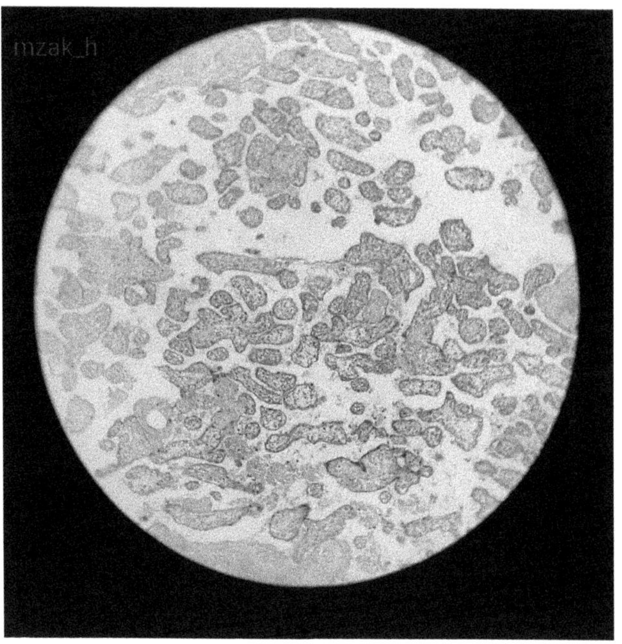

PLACENTA

Umbilical cord

- umbilical cord is covered by amnion membrane

- matrix of umbilical cord is formed by wharton's jelly
- Two umbilical arteries and one umbilical vein can observe

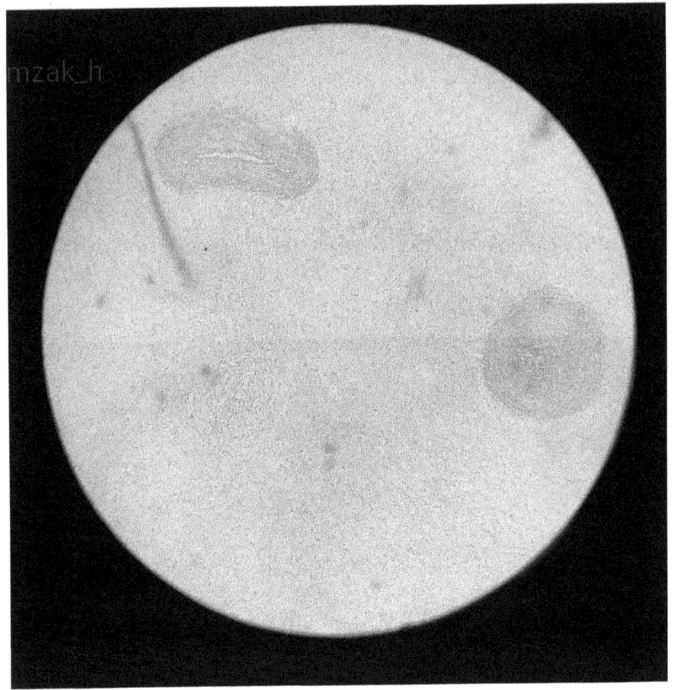

UMBILICAL CORD

• • •

CHAPTER XXVI

VASCULAR TISSUE

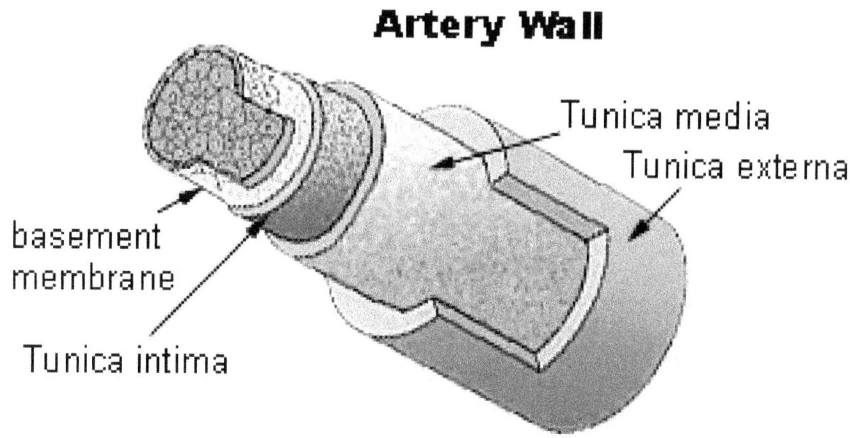

IMAGE: ARTERIAL WALL (IMG CREDIT; Illu artery)

All blood vessels has following layers

1. Tunica intima : consists of endothelium, sub endothelial- connective tissue and internal elastic lamina
2. Tunica media : It is composed of connective tissue fibres and smooth muscles. It is separated from tunica adventitia by 'external elastic lamina'
3. Tunica Adventitia : composed of connective tissue. Posses" Vasa vasorum" and "nervi vasorum"

Large/elastic artery(eg:aorta)

- presence of many elastic fibres in "tunica media". Smooth muscle content is less
- internal elastic lamina is not prominent

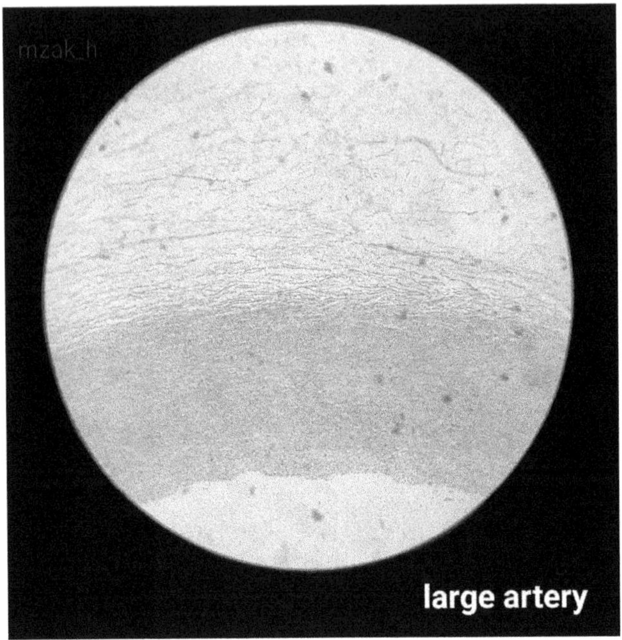

H&E SLIDE LARGE ARTERY

Medium sized /muscular artery (eg:palmar.A)

- Tunica media contains abundance of smooth muscles and few elastic fibres
- prominent internal elastic lamina

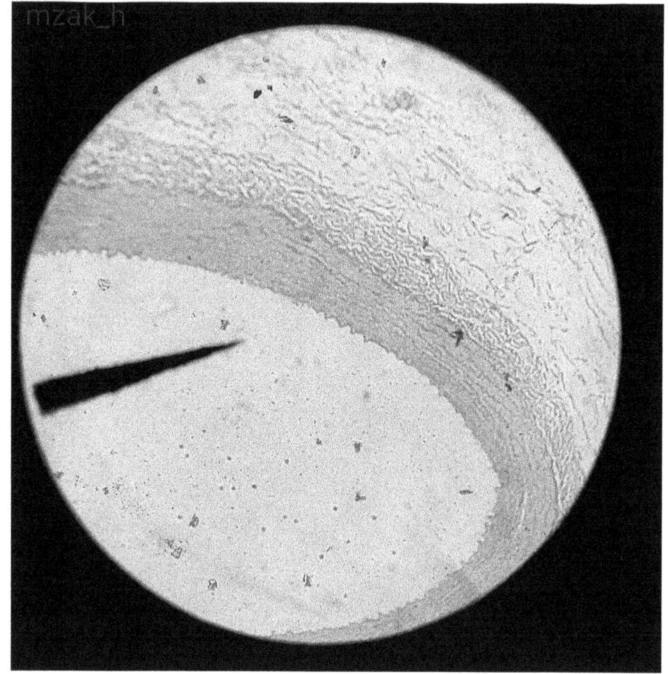

H&E SLIDE MEDIUM SIZED ARTERY

Large vein(eg:svc)

- Thick tunica adventitia with longitudinal bundles of smooth muscles
- poorly developed tunica media

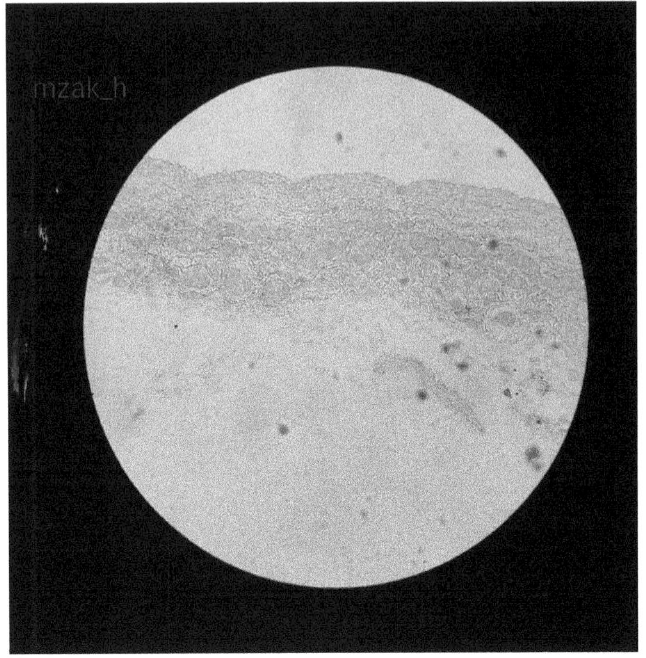

H&E SLIDE LARGE SIZED VEIN

Medium sized vein

- characterized by collapsed lumen
- tunica media with few smooth muscle fibres and Elastic fibers

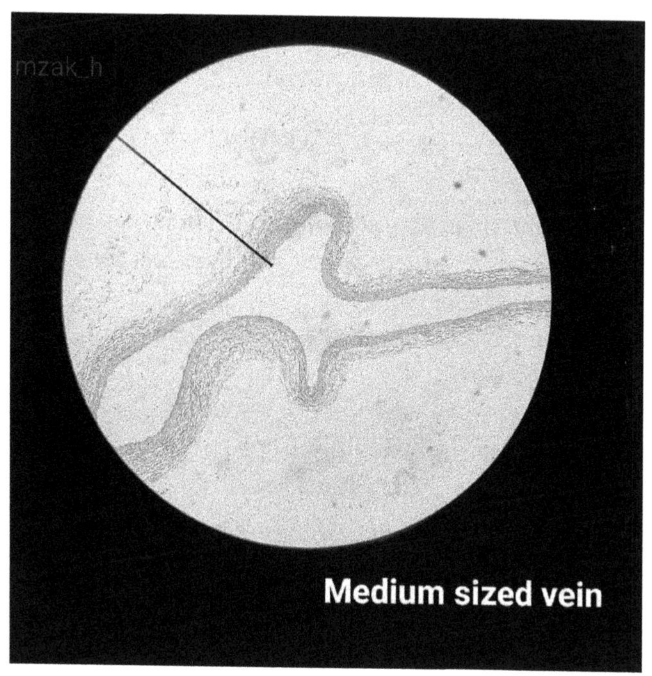

H&E SLIDE MEDIUM SIZED VEIN

• • •

CHAPTER XXVII

BONE

- The structural unit of a compact bone is osteon or haversian system
- Osteons are made up of concentric lamellae of bone matrix with a central canal called haversian canal
- Within the bone matrix there are spaces called lacunae, which are occupied by osteocytes
- Between the Osteons we can observe remnants of previous concentric lamellae called Interstitial lamellae
- Each osteons are transversely connected by volkmann's canal

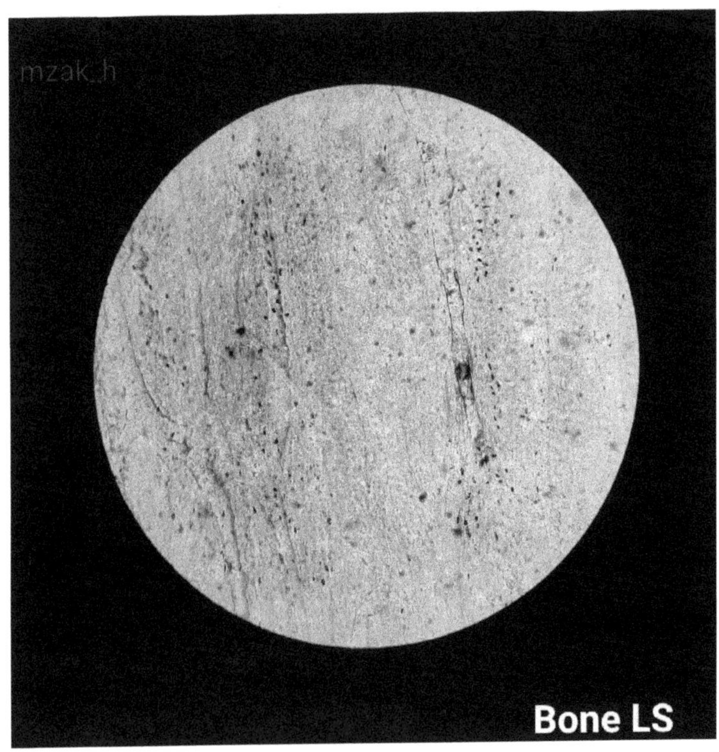

H&E SLIDE BONE L.S

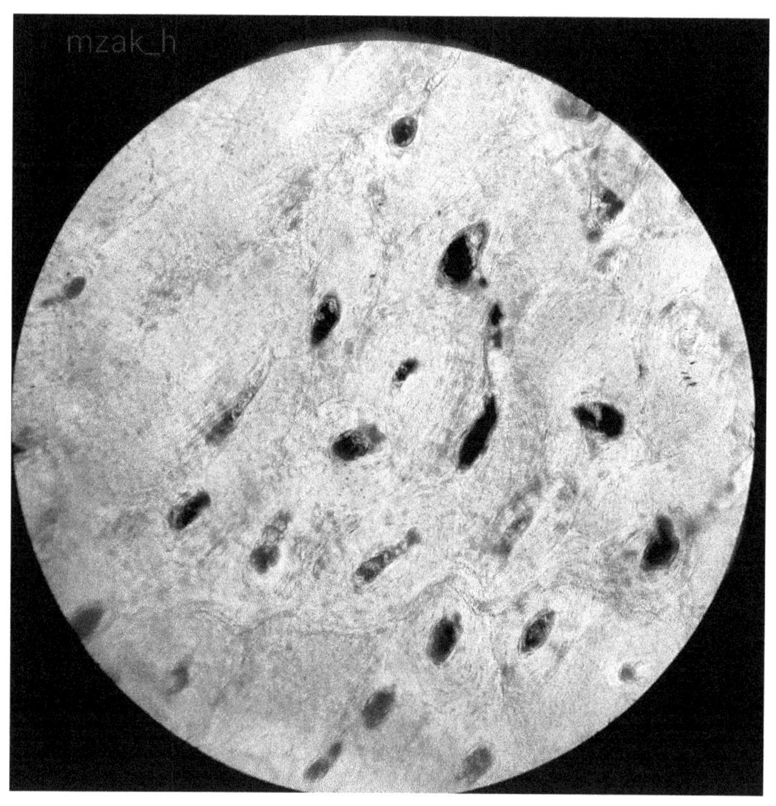

H&E SLIDE BONE T.S

• • •

www.ingramcontent.com/pod-product-compliance
Ingram Content Group UK Ltd.
Pitfield, Milton Keynes, MK11 3LW, UK
UKHW021924190726
13853UKWH00002B/834

9 798886 840155